Dorothy G. Kline
56 Park Street
Brandon, VT 05733

THE
FAMILY HERBAL

A Guide to Natural Health Care for
Yourself and Your Children from Europe's
Leading Herbalists

BARBARA & PETER THEISS

Healing Arts Press
Rochester, Vermont

Healing Arts Press
One Park Street
Rochester, Vermont 05767

Copyright © 1989, 1993 by Barbara and Peter Theiss

All rights reserved. No part of this book may be reproduced or utilized in any form or by any means, electronic or mechanical, including photocopying, recording, or by any information storage and retrieval system, without permission in writing from the publisher.

Note to the reader: This book is intended as an informational guide. The remedies, approaches, and techniques described herein are meant to supplement, and not to be a substitute for, professional medical care or treatment. They should not be used to treat a serious ailment without prior consultation with a qualified healthcare professional.

Library of Congress Cataloging-in-Publication Data
Theiss, Barbara.
    The family herbal : a guide to natural health care for yourself and your children from Europe's leading herbalists / Barbara and Peter Theiss. —Rev. ed.
        p.   cm.
    Includes bibliographical references and index.
    ISBN 0-89281-484-5
    I. Herbs—Therapeutic use. I. Theiss, Peter. II. Title.
RM666.H33T45   1993
615'.321—dc20   93-13856
                                                                      CIP

Printed and bound in Hong Kong

10 9 8 7 6 5 4 3 2 1

Text design by Charlotte Tyler

Healing Arts Press is a division of Inner Traditions International

Distributed to the book trade in the United States by American International
    Distribution Corporation (AIDC)
Distributed to the book trade in Canada by Publishers Group West (PGW),
    Montreal West, Quebec
Distributed to the health food trade in Canada by Alive Books, Toronto and
    Vancouver
Distributed to the book trade in the United Kingdom by Deep Books, London
Distributed to the book trade in Australia by Millennium Books, Newtown,
    N. S. W.

CONTENTS

ACKNOWLEDGMENTS

It may interest our readers to know that this book was *not* first written in German (our native language) and then translated into English. Rather, the German- and English-language editions of the book were actually two distinct works, written at the same time, yet as separate efforts. We wanted *The Family Herbal* to be a conversation between ourselves and you, the reader, and no mere translation would have been able to express the essence of what we wanted to say—or the way we wanted to say it—to our English-speaking friends.

We are deeply grateful to the women and men of Inner Traditions for their caring, competent efforts. They were a joy to work with, and they made the tasks of writing, designing, checking details, editing, and production a smooth and rewarding process for all of us. Our sincere thanks go especially to the firm but gentle touch of Leslie Colket and Susan Davidson, who managed the project. Special thanks also to our copyeditor, Karen Ready, whose job was to make the book better, and who did that and more.

We have reserved our greatest thanks for our dear friend John Fogg, who helped us to write the text for the American edition. John struggled to marry incompatible computers, only to witness them eat entire chapters. He pored over six different dictionaries to find the precise words we wanted to use. His dedication throughout to accuracy as well as underlying meaning, his patience, and his willingness to pursue details beyond any reasonable expectations were a constant gift. We believe this gift has been passed on to you as well.

In the face of difficulties and challenges, it was John's remarkable sense of humor that kept us going. We fondly remember how often his calls and faxes would refresh us even in the midst of dull office routine. A major portion of the editing and rewriting was accomplished while John was a guest at our home in Homburg/Saar. The fun and laughter that filled our writing studio on the third floor were such that our thirteen-year-old son, Jonas, simply could not believe that we were actually *working!*

Our heartfelt thanks to John for his contributions to this book.

PREFACE
TO THE REVISED EDITION

Since the first edition of *The Family Herbal* was published, the scientific discussion of medicinal herbs has continued and has presented many new findings. We too have learned more by receiving and answering hundreds of letters from readers all over the world. In addition, of course, our personal experience has also widened, for life does not stand still.

For this revised edition, every bit of information in the book has been carefully checked against the newest available knowledge, and changes have been made wherever necessary. Comfrey (*Symphytum officinale*) is the only herb we have dropped; the results of new research have seriously questioned its safety for both internal and external application. Although there are great differences in comfrey depending upon its country of origin, and although the scientists involved in comfrey research hope that it will be possible to breed new varieties without the potentially dangerous pyrrolizidine alkaloids, we deemed it wiser for the present to omit this herb from our book. Instead, we have incorporated ginseng, which is not only a best-seller in the marketplace but also one of the most thoroughly researched medicinal plants.

A new chapter, "Create your own herb garden," is intended to inspire and instruct our readers in the practical realization of their wish to grow their own herbs for both culinary and health care use.

To make self-medication easier for the reader, we have changed all measurements from grams to parts. We hope this will now eliminate all stumbling blocks for those who want to personally blend their teas and tinctures.

Last but not least, a list of recommended readings, a bibliography, a more accurate plant index, a table of plant parts, and a comprehensive therapeutic index make this book more handy for the reader who seeks specific advice in a particular situation.

It has been a joy for us to see that so far 300,000 copies of *The Family Herbal* have been sold and that the book has been published in nine different languages, with the tenth and eleventh to follow in 1993. Furthermore, it fills us with great satisfaction that since the beginning of our "herbal preaching" some twenty years ago, the attitude toward herbal remedies and natural ways of healing in general has changed quite remarkably. It looks as though these outstanding benefactors of humanity are well on their way to regaining the respect and recognition they deserve.

❧ 1 ❧

THE PURPOSE OF OUR BOOK

We have written this book because we know that when medicinal herbs again become an integral part of daily life for us all, our world will be a healthier, happier, and more peaceful place for our children and our children's children.

One hundred years ago, it was customary for a housewife in Europe, and in America as well, to prepare most of the medications her family would need for the upcoming year. She would select herbs that grew in her garden and add others that the family had gathered in the surrounding fields and forests. Linden flowers were picked and dried for treating colds during the winter season. Calendula ointment was made fresh from bright summer blossoms, to be used for healing cuts and scrapes. Bitter roots were dug in the fall and put into spirits to create elixirs that would soothe upset stomachs and help digestion. Harvesting the medicinal plants that grew in the immediate area, processing and preserving them, was just as natural as "putting up" vegetables or canning fruits from the garden and backyard orchard.

In the course of the changes that have taken place in our modern world, in our family structures, our work and social relationships, our diets and lifestyles—changes in every aspect of life over the past one hundred years—we have left the preparation of medicinal remedies completely in the hands of pharmacists and drug companies. We have certainly lost the experience, the knowledge, and—what is most sad of all—the personal initiative we may have once had to heal ourselves. The tragedy is that doctors, pharmacists, and pharmaceutical manufacturers alike have also forgotten the art and science of medicinal herbs. Blinded by the huge profit possibilities offered by the medical establishment, many health care professionals dismiss the idea of natural healing with herbs. Not until an alarming number of these synthetic pharmaceutical products had been in use for decades and had been shown to be toxic time bombs did people begin to remember the safety and effectiveness of "good old" healing herbs.

In 1909, Alexander Tschirch, the farsighted cofounder of the science of pharmaceutical biology (which—unlike pharmaceutical chemistry—is involved with the study of medicinal plants), said, "Not until medical science has gotten indigestion from synthetic chemical medications and has experimented with all the organs of laboratory animals, will it return to man's oldest remedies, medicinal plants." Today we have begun to do just that.

We are literally undergoing a revolution. People are no longer willing to heedlessly take cardiovascular stimulants, sleeping pills, and painkillers. We have come to question the great variety of drugs prescribed by the medical establishment. Each one of us has observed in ourselves, our family, or our closest friends how the use of synthetic chemicals to treat the symptoms of diseases and disorders at best only helps in the short term. We have seen and felt for ourselves the serious side effects of these powerful "man-made" chemicals. Many of us, regrettably, have experienced the debilitating effect these artificial drugs have on our body's natural defense mechanisms.

What a joy it is to see so many people again fighting colds with warm herbal-essence vapors; stimulating their circulation with an invigorating hot foot bath; rubbing their aching joints with homemade oil of St. Johnswort; and enjoying a delicious, calming cup of herbal tea every evening. Herbs are excellent agents for self-medication. They can help relieve countless, everyday complaints in a gentle, natural way without the specter of serious side effects. However, it would be inaccurate and irresponsible to claim that remedies based on herbs have no side effects. Whenever there is any known side effect, we will mention it along with the description of the respective herb in the following chapters.

Basically speaking, any health problem should be responded to quickly, so as to not give it a chance to become established in our bodies. It must not be given the opportunity to "take hold." Therefore, it is imperative that we react promptly to any feeling of indisposition or pain. Please bear in mind that a feeling of pain is nothing other than an alarm signal; it is the body's way of announcing that something is amiss and requires your attention. Everyone has had the experience of warding off an illness by catching it just when it was starting to "rear its ugly head." This should always be your objective. This is also where medicinal herbs are most effective: when you feel you are coming down with a cold; when you have a slight scratchy feeling in your throat; when your tendons are starting to ache because you have overexercised; when a bloated feeling heralds a digestive problem; or when insomnia signals that you are under too much stress. These are all examples of the problems that most healthy individuals experience at one time or another and that occur in every normal family. It is a blessing to know that something can be done about them right now, instead of waiting a week and then going to the doctor because you have become seriously ill.

Herbs aren't just for minor illnesses either. Chronic conditions, such as arthritis or cardiac weakness, as well as recurring functional disorders, such as bladder infection or gastritis, can be successfully treated with herbs. Long-term herbal therapy is quite often very useful in such cases. Furthermore, the disorders of old age that are typically found in our culture, such as arthritis or high blood pressure, are actually better treated with natural remedies than with synthetic medications. Otherwise, high quantities of harmful residues from foodstuffs and medications accumulate in the organism of elderly persons and of themselves inhibit the proper functioning of the organs.

Medicinal plants are excellent for counteracting disturbances of the autonomic nervous system, which are constantly on the increase in industrialized countries because of our unnatural, stress-ridden way of life. Here the harmonizing effects of herbs are revealed, for unlike synthetic sleeping agents, laxatives, "uppers," "downers," and so on, herbs rarely have undesirable side effects and are hardly ever habit-forming.

Finally, medicinal herbs also serve as excellent secondary therapeutic agents that as a rule can safely and effectively be combined with many primary forms of therapy. In some cases it is extremely useful to combine treatment by a strong chemical drug with a blood-purifying tea or elixir, so that the body can be induced to excrete the alien and heavily toxic substances as quickly as possible.

Apart from all these therapeutic possibilities, we cannot emphasize enough the preventative effect of medicinal herbs. Prevention means cleaning out, purifying, and detoxifying on a regular basis—even daily. In the tradition of herbology there are so-called blood purification cures that are undertaken each spring and fall. This practice of regular purification has been proved to be highly effective, as shown by the latest clinical findings in connection with fasting cures and intestinal flushing. This is the secret of those rare individuals who are healthy in body and spirit as well as active in old age: regular purification and fasting cures! (More on this subject will be covered in chapter 5.)

Our book is especially intended for families, for fathers and mothers who want to care for the health problems and day-to-day aches and pains of their children and family members by using medications that are as natural as possible. Of course, this doesn't mean your doctor is to be avoided at any cost, but an attempt should first be made to treat unwanted conditions with the gentle remedies offered by Mother Nature, to nip them in the bud wherever possible, and even to prevent them from occurring at all.

Although this work provides precise descriptions and illustrations of many of the medicinal herbs we believe to be the most important, it is not intended to be a textbook for the identification and exact study of individual medicinal plants. Even within any one particular geographic or climatic zone—northern Europe, for example—there are several thousand different herbs to be considered. Our book is intended to offer the beginner a very practical introduction to healing with medicinal herbs—which simply means doing the right thing for a minor bladder infection in your child, treating your own finger burned by a hot pan, or soothing your baby's chafed bottom.

We have purposely limited ourselves to forty medicinal herbs that we call basic herbs. These herbs are indigenous to Germany, our native country, yet all of them grow within the various climatic zones of the

United States. They can easily be found and collected, if one has a good knowledge of gathering herbs, or they may be purchased throughout the world in natural pharmacies, natural or health food stores, and herb shops. (A number of fine mail order businesses now offer quality herbs as well; see the list of suppliers on page 269.) These forty basic herbs have proved to be the most successful, best-studied, and in our opinion most effective herbs for the respective symptoms and areas of indication. We have described every herb and accompanied each entry with a full-color illustration. The application is always a combination of traditional knowledge handed down through our rich herbal heritage, the latest scientific findings, and our own personal experience. Information on effect and administration is based on the latest research contained in plant monographs published by a special department of the Federal German Health Office, the so-called Evaluative Compilation Commission E for Phytotherapy (Aufbereitungskommission E für Phytotherapie), compiled in year-long collaboration with institutions of higher learning and leading research laboratories. In addition, we have chosen basic herbs that can be used to treat almost all cases of minor ill-health occurring in your family. Finally, we have added to the list several additional herbs that we find helpful or necessary to round off some of the prescribed formulas.

Our book is concerned with the practical application of medicinal plants for your family's health care. We believe it to be extremely important that the ancient traditional knowledge of healing herbs return to use in the family. Children can almost always be helped by natural remedies, assuming they are born in a state of relatively good health. Their afflictions, like their bodies and minds, are generally not as intractable as those of adults; the child's organism still responds much more sensitively to minute stimuli and still possesses a virtually inexhaustible regenerative power. (This particularly applies to babies, of course; indeed, medicinal herbs are a boon not only during birth, but during pregnancy too.) If our children learn early in their lives to help themselves by using herbs, they will continue to do so as adults, and they will in turn pass this knowledge on to their children as well.

It goes without saying that these tips and instructions are also useful for single people. The only difference is that these persons generally have only themselves to look after, and are not usually confronted by the great variety of complaints faced by the parents of growing families. Basically speaking, it is vital for everyone to know about herbs and how best to use them.

Once you discover how successful you can be at treating yourself and others and how enjoyable it is to use medicinal herbs, you are apt to become increasingly curious about the plants themselves, their individual characteristics and unique healing qualities. We urge you to refer to other herbals for more information on the way herbs work and how to recognize them in the wild. (See, for example, David Hoffmann's *The Herbal Handbook: A User's Guide to Medical Herbalism,* Rochester, Vt., 1989, or the classic textbook *Herbal Medicine,* by Rudolf Fritz Weiss, M.D., Heidelberg, 1988.) Another way to involve yourself with herbs is by collecting them, harvesting, processing, and preserving them, and preparing them for use. You may also want to add a medicinal plant section to your own garden. Libraries and bookstores are filled with many engaging and informative books offering advice on all of these subjects.

The amount of information available on natural health care methods and healing with medicinal plants and herbs is extraordinarily large. Yet this material covers only a very small part of the plant kingdom. There are about 380,000 species of plants in our world, of which 260,000 belong to the group of so-called higher plants; of these, only 10 percent at most have been studied to any significant extent. Analyzing the rest will occupy scientists for generations to come.

❦ 2 ❦

OUR OWN STORY

*The greatest events are not our loudest but rather
our quietest hours.*

Friedrich Nietzsche

BARBARA'S STORY

My interest in herbs began during a period in my life when I had a need
to withdraw from the world, to self-reflect and meditate. I had just passed
my college preparatory graduation examination with flying colors
and had decided to study German philology because of my deep love
of literature and philosophy. I was quite disillusioned and frustrated
to discover how dry, spiritless, and seemingly without purpose the university degree program was. This realization, coupled with some increasing physical and psychological difficulties I was experiencing, propelled
me in a completely new life direction, one that I had never considered
before.

I learned to cure myself through the practice of yoga and breathing
therapy, and I began to become conscious of nutrition as well. Soon I
was so fascinated by all these new activities that I chose to drop my
university studies and turn instead to healing. I studied breathing therapy
with several expert teachers and completed a program of study to obtain my license as a Heilpraktiker, or "healing practitioner" (a title not

7

officially recognized in the United States, with training and requirements much like a Doctor of Chiropractic, yet covering more fields of study, such as herbology, acupuncture, and homeopathy).

At the beginning of this period in my life, I would seek relaxation and inspiration by making weekend visits to Kochel am See, a picturesque village in the Lower Alps of Bavaria. I spent hours and days on end in self-reflective peace and solitude in my father's hunting lodge, which was located on the edge of an isolated moorland at the foot of the mountains. It was here, amidst the breathtaking beauty of unspoiled nature, that my interest in medicinal plants began to awaken.

I bought my first book about herbs and took it with me on all my quiet walks and hikes up into the mountains. I collected, compared, smelled, tasted, and took notes, fascinated by the possibilities for healing that lay hidden in these marvelous plants. In this simple patch of God's green earth, medicine was growing right out of the ground: wherever I trod I was stepping on precious healing substances from Nature's Pharmacy. Filled with happiness at making this discovery, I continued studying until I was familiar with the majority of herbs and medicinal plants that grew in the region—and there were no fewer than several hundred. I collected and dried them, experimented with different formulas and preparations, and tried them all out on myself, my family, and my patients as well. I had come upon an inconceivable wealth of healing possibilities, and my interest kept on growing in leaps and bounds.

In the summer of 1972, I was back in my favorite place taking a two-week long fasting cure. Fasting always heightens my senses and even makes me a little clairvoyant; indeed, it makes me feel closer to heaven. This time, I had a clear and powerful vision of how people could really heal themselves with herbs. I saw how sick people have to seek out in a truly spiritual manner the plant that can cure them, how they must approach the plant with reverence and ask for help, whereupon the herb will offer up its healing energy for them. I saw myself as an intermediary who would show sick people what to do. And I saw myself—actually my spirit, my true nature and purpose—as a healer. Anyone who has had a similar experience and has felt just how far back our roots reach into our unconscious past will know what an inner strength and powerful sense of purpose this gave me.

PETER'S STORY

When I met Barbara, I had already completed my pharmacist's degree and was working on my doctoral dissertation. I was fortunate to have completed practical training in a large, versatile pharmacy in Frankfurt, in which all types of ointments, tablets, capsules, and other preparations were made in the old, traditional manner. This enabled me to learn the pharmacist's art from scratch.

At this point my thirst for knowledge drove me to become active in research. I wanted to know exactly what effects medications, and in particular narcotics, have on the human body and consciousness. I spent most of my time at work in the laboratory of the Max Planck Institute for Psychiatry in Munich, where I made tablets containing morphine and experimented, testing how the pain-relieving drug altered the behavior of rats. I studied neurotransmitters and the function of the organs within a single nerve-ending cell and discussed my findings at international congresses. I was well on my way to becoming a successful scientist.

When Barbara, who was at that time my yoga teacher, took me along to the mountains on an herb expedition, I was surprised to discover that although I had heard of these herbs during my studies and had even identified botanical specimens in examinations, all I really knew about medicinal plants was their Latin nomenclature and active ingredients. Barbara and I both developed a keen interest in the remarkable variety of healing effects and various formulas, mixtures, and preparations. We both loved the wild mountain countryside, the moorland marshes, and the meadows with their health-bringing medicinal plants, and we never returned from an excursion without a collection of fragrant, aromatic herbs. It was at that time that Barbara and I started our lives together.

During the final year that I worked on my dissertation, I took on a post as the head of production in a small company located in Munich, the manufacturer of a whole array of herbal medications. This was a major period of learning for me, a time when I became more deeply acquainted with the manufacture of herbal medications.

This period in my life proved to be a very trying one. Our first child,

Jonas, arrived, and the realities of family life required immediate change and adaptation. It was during this time that my father repeated an offer he had made once before: that I take over his pharmacy in Homburg/ Saar, my hometown.

Barbara and I were in a great dilemma. Our conscience would not allow us to sell people chemical-based medications, e.g. painkillers, sleeping drugs, or antibiotics, unless they were faced with a life-threatening situation. Yet the working regulations for pharmacies required that all of these powerful medications be kept in stock and that they be available to dispense to patients when prescribed by a physician. Night after night of soul-searching discussions finally led us to the difficult decision to take over the pharmacy despite our reservations. We felt it was best to take a stand for our high ideals and become personally involved.

It was difficult to part with our lifestyle in Munich, our friends and the things we loved so much to do. In Saarland, the state in which Homburg is located, we felt like lonely pioneers with our way of thinking. But we plunged into work at the pharmacy. To celebrate our first Christmas in Homburg, six months later, we gave each customer an attractive jar of herbal tea with a tag bearing the proverb "Better to light a candle than to complain about the darkness." Barbara, who was known from the start for her artistic window decorations, carried out this theme by lighting candles in the display windows of the pharmacy, which is located prominently on the market square in the heart of town.

Inside the pharmacy things were turned upside down and inside out, remodeled, and reorganized. Every day I stood behind the counter in my white coat and bet with myself whether or not we would succeed that day in making the sales quota we required. My hitherto latent business acumen was literally forced into the light by daily practice. I waited personally on every customer who came in and advised him or her to the best of my knowledge and belief. As my advice obviously tended in the direction of more natural medications, I recommended many herbs and homeopathic preparations as well. And the customers really appreciated it! They saw that we were not merely interested in filling expensive prescriptions but were genuinely concerned with their problems, their symptoms and illnesses, as well as with the unwanted side effects many complained about from the prescribed medications they were taking.

Barbara worked in the background, thought up marketing concepts, and decorated the pharmacy accordingly. She designed informational brochures and created sales campaigns that we carried out together. We also began to prepare a series of lectures about herbs using color slides. In the evening after work, I traveled through the area giving talks and lectures to such diverse groups as garden clubs, Kneipp associations (followers of the teachings of the German naturopath Sebastian Kneipp), and local women's clubs.

After about two years, more and more people from the surrounding country and towns were making the pilgrimage to Homburg in order to purchase their herbal medications from "Dr. Theiss, the pharmacist." Barbara led herb walks and nature excursions in the spring and summer, which always turned most of the participants into collectors and users of herbs. Gradually we came to have a very enthusiastic group of students and customers.

In the winter of 1976 I developed twenty-five different medicinal herb tea mixtures, ranging from a sedative tea to a tonic tea for a variety of complaints, which we registered and sold in our pharmacy as specialties of the house. Many of these teas were enthusiastically received from the start.

One day an elderly lady came into the pharmacy carrying a formula written on a tattered piece of paper. She asked us to make a mixture of the herbs and substances it listed—a very difficult task, as it turned out, because the list included extremely rare ingredients. In my ambition to provide whatever was requested, I went to a great deal of trouble to recreate the exact formula and finally succeeded in preparing the elixir for the lady. When she came in to pick it up she said, "Please make up another liter for my neighbor. This is something very special; I am positive you will sell a lot of it." She turned out to be right, for although I did not know it at the time, this formula turned out to be the recipe for Swedish Bitters, a remarkable elixir that has changed the lives of thousands of people—especially ours!

After four years, sales at the pharmacy had doubled; whereas prescription medicines had previously made up 80 percent of sales, they now made up only 50 percent. The other half of our sales was made up of over-the-counter medicinal agents, which included body care items, cosmetics, and dietetic products as well as herbal teas and preparations. The ratio of 50:50 is most unusual for a pharmacy in Germany, as the business mainly serves to dispense prescription medicines. Yet our customers demonstrated over and over again that they preferred medicinal herb preparations. This is even more remarkable when you understand that our customers were often paying for these herbal products out of their own pockets. In Germany, where everyone is covered by national health insurance, the chemical-based medicines that are prescribed by physicians are almost always paid for completely by the health plan, whereas herbal medicines and naturopathic remedies are not always covered.

Our interest in old herb books, traditional formulas, and natural healing methods propelled us further along in our studies. The wisdom of the ancient alchemists held great fascination for Barbara and me, and it was on account of this interest that we traveled to the United States for the first time. It was here, in the New World, that we met the teacher Frater Albertus, with whom we studied the healing secrets of the Old World. One direct result of all this was Barbara's first writing on the relationship between herbs and astrological influences, that is, the association of various herbs to the planets and how those influences can serve to guide us in the selection and preparation of many wonderful herbal remedies. For many years now, Barbara has studied the works of the ancient alchemists—for example the views of Paracelsus on medicinal herbs, and in particular his doctrine of signatures.

My entrepreneurial spirit was not yet satisfied. I needed still another outlet to expand my field of activity. So in 1979, Barbara and I founded Naturwaren GmbH, a company involved in the manufacture of remedies and preparations based on medicinal herbs that could be sold by other pharmacies as well as our own. Barbara required that all the packaging and promotional materials for Naturwaren be artfully designed and be a genuine expression of the high quality and true spirit of these simple, natural medications.

Throughout Europe and the world, the "comeback" of herbology was now in full swing. We called it the Herbal Renaissance. As a result of the sale of millions of copies of *Health from God's Pharmacy* (Steyr, Austria, 1984), a work by the great Austrian herbalist Maria Treben, untold numbers of people read about the healing power of herbs and began to try them for themselves. Swedish Bitters (a precursor of the formula given in Chapter 8), which was highly acclaimed and recommended in the book, became an instant hit.

The triumphant advance of herbal remedies and preparations was achieved by people like you and me, the host of men and women who have suffered illnesses and have sought an alternative system of treatment. It was certainly not promoted by the scientific or medical establishment—the doctors, pharmacists, and professional medical people. Indeed, my fellow pharmacists resisted the new wave with all their might. After all, they had learned at the university that herbology was an assortment of folklore reaching far back into the Dark Ages without any real scientific basis. In other words, pharmacists—apart from a few exceptions—were generally adverse to our concept of natural healing, and it wasn't until they saw the brisk business to be done with these items that they hesitatingly changed their attitude.

It was during this period that we met and became friends with Maria Treben. Barbara and I would go out with her after the lectures that she held before audiences of thousands of eager listeners, and talk about herbs and share our experiences. Through Maria and her husband we became acquainted with several beautiful spots in Austria where the most marvelous and rarest herbs were to be found. We went with them to search for arnica and club moss, for example, which was a special experience.

Maria would tell us stories about her early years, and related how she had survived during the war on only mushrooms, berries, and herbs. She told us how she herself discovered the healing power of herbs and how she continually expanded her knowledge and experience concerning them. What has sustained the bond between us through the many years is our mutual, deeply felt love of nature and our reverence for its gifts. We had all realized that we need only call graciously on nature to help ourselves compensate for our deficiencies and shortcomings to become truly healthy and happy again.

I never really had a care for the future success of our business. As more and more people became interested in the herbal preparations we were offering, I knew we would expand simply because our satisfied customers would generate more new customers. My job was to do the business in the best way: creating new products, making changes to help us become more effective in our work, and so on. Although I had entertained bold dreams that we would eventually become an international company, I never harbored any real intention to do business in the United States.

Yet Barbara and I were attracted to America as if by magic, and in

1979 we first traveled to the United States to study. We soon recognized that in comparison with Europeans, Americans had very little knowledge about herbs and their uses, perhaps because the break with tradition had been more abrupt and more far-reaching in the States. However, Americans responded to our ideas with their proverbial openness and enthusiasm. In 1984 a new test of our entrepreneurial spirit began with the founding of our American company NatureWorks, Inc. Since then, we have developed a genuine love for the many wonderful people we have met and worked with in the United States.

❧ 3 ❧

NATURE'S PHARMACY VERSUS MAN'S PHARMACY

The Lord hath created medicines out of the earth; and the wise will not abhor them.

Ben Sira 38:4

In the sixth century B.C., during the Buddha's lifetime, there lived in India a man by the name of Jivaka. For seven years, he received instruction from his master, a renowned physician. One day, he asked his master when he would be allowed to treat people himself. Instead of answering Jivaka's question, the master advised him, "Go out into the surrounding area and bring back everything that possesses a healing power." Jivaka set off, returning three days later. "The task you gave me is impossible," he told his master. "I cannot bring back everything I have found that has healing power. It would be too much to carry. For everything in nature has curative power, every plant has healing properties, as does every animal and every mineral." Jivaka thus proved his qualification as a healer and in time became one of India's greatest physicians.

The truth of Jivaka's discovery has been recognized by the great natural healers of all ages and cultures. They all have a basic trust of nature. They stand in the knowledge that everything in the universe is connected, and they see individual people as a part and a reflection of the cosmos. If disease can occur as the material precipitation of disorder and lack of harmony, then somewhere must exist the power and energy to transform this disorder back to harmony and health. An inner understanding of cosmic analogies leads the natural healer to the same conclusion as Paracelsus, the master herbalist of the sixteenth century, who expressed it in his famous saying, "Against every ill there is an herb that grows."

In earlier days, the healer was always a priest or priestess as well, for the wise, the inspired, the magician, mystic, or shaman possessed an enlightened viewpoint of what his or her fellows experienced as disease. Such knowledge was based on his or her uncommon familiarity with the world of the spirit or the planes of higher energies. It was the healer-priest who knew about medicinal plants and who advised the sick to assimilate the healing energy and power of herbs. Hippocrates, Galen, Hildegard of Bingen, Albertus Magnus, Paracelsus, Sebastian Kneipp, and Johann Künzle are known in Europe, but innumerable men and women from every culture on this earth have served their people as shamans or healer-priests.

It is our opinion that a fundamental trust in nature established on spiritual and philosophical understanding is still a prerequisite today for anyone wishing to delve into the depths of (natural) healing. Where people have lost respect for life and where there is no simple wonder at the beauty of a flower or the invisible life force of a seed, there can be no foundation for herbal healing. We highly recommend the book *The Secret Life of Plants,* by Peter Tompkins and Christopher Bird (New York, 1984), for those who as a result of our artificial way of life have not been able to develop this trust through their own feelings. It will help you to understand—on the intellectual level, at least—with what wonderful sensibility and intelligence plants are endowed.

Today, as we slowly emerge from the nightmare of an artificial world of chemically controlled body machines and set about renewing our understanding of what our earth means to us and what we owe it, the words of Paracelsus are just as valid as they were in the sixteenth century: "Your meadows and pastures shall be your pharmacies."

Every era has its problems and its concerns. One of the important missions we must accept is to reveal, verify, and correct the traditional beliefs we hold. Because of the intimate relationship between healing and spiritual concepts, some of the things we find in old books are simply not comprehensible; they cry out to be freed from superstition, mystification, and exaggeration before we can make practical use of them. We are quite correct to test herbs for their healing qualities by the modern means we have available today. We must subject herbs to scientific testing methods employing complicated high-technology instruments and apparatus, even if it is true that this process has its inherent problems. Our scientific methods of investigation have been developed using mechanistic-logical thought concepts and abstract premises. Yet all too often these methods fail to comprehend the life principle, the true nature and complexity of either a plant or the human organism. What is needed today is an understanding that fuses our keenly developed twentieth-century analytical minds with the profound spiritual wisdom of past ages. The modern scientific study of herbs and medicinal plants, which will replace the imprecise and vague areas known as "herbal" and "folk" medicine, is the newly named field of phytotherapy (a term derived from Greek to refer to the treatment of diseases and disorders by plants).

There is the direction of strict, analytical science, which regards the plant as a more or less impure product, whose active principle must be detected, analyzed, and tested. The aim is to isolate this ingredient from the plant. Scientists from this school of thought are of the opinion that this is the only way to obtain objective pharmacological data, especially with regard to sustainable and repeatable effects. One of their aims is the standardization of the active agents in both the plants themselves and the medications made from them. Variations and irregularities in the medicinal plants are a thorn in the flesh of such scientists, and they avoid mixing herbs together because of the difficulties this makes for precise and proper analysis.

The opposite point of view regards the plant as synergistic, a complex composition of active ingredients and accompanying substances whose whole makes up more than the sum of its individual parts. The reduction of herbs to isolated active ingredients is regarded as a limitation of possibilities, which actually inhibits the real healing potential. In the eyes of such scientists, the whole plant should come into action in its entirety. This school of thought also accepts the experiences obtained in practical application—in addition to the pure analysis of active ingredients—as "evidence" for the effectivity of an herb. The results of practical experience lead these men and women to advocate the blending of various medicinal herbs together.

We make no secret of the fact that we are full-blooded exponents of the latter, holistic principle, and we like to quote the illustration of "the symphony of active principles" created by our pharmacist colleague Mannfried Pahlow. When a large orchestra plays a symphony, each instrument, even the most seemingly unimportant, must contribute its unique and special sound at the proper moment. So too, it is fundamentally important for the effects of medicinal herbs that each and every ingredient be present and "in tune"—even when we as yet have no idea of the role each part may play. Analytical science, which tears everything apart, has too great a tendency to deny the principles of other systems merely because it cannot explain them or does not know enough about them. Sufficient proof already exists that accompanying substances such as minerals, vitamins, enzymes, trace minerals, amino acids, chlorophyll, aromas, and coloring matter can act as catalysts for the so-called active ingredient in any healing substance. In fact, they may be the very things that make it possible for the active agent to act at all! Isn't nature with all its complex biochemistry wiser than we who possess only a fragmentary knowledge of her mysterious and infinite interactions?

Against this range of differing opinions we want to define our own standpoint and methods as follows: We take tradition very seriously—tradition that is based on experience stretching back for thousands of years. We respect and seek those intuitive insights that recognize and honor plants as our magical partners in life. We make use of science, as well as modern chemical and pharmaceutical methods, in order to meet the requirements of the law and the marketplace. Each of these seemingly disparate approaches helps us to check and balance each of the others. This is because we have learned not to rely on just one method. However, our most basic principle is that of holistic medicine, which perceives the human being as a functioning whole of body, mind, and spirit, an integral and never-separated part of our living earth and universe.

From humankind's experience of industrialization over the last hundred years, we have learned—or should have learned—that valuable nutrition can be turned into harmful junk food and harmonizing healing medicaments into dangerous poisons and narcotic drugs, if we rob them of their natural accompaniments, "denaturalize" and "industrialize" them. Any chemical component has a more dramatic, definitive effect when it is isolated and concentrated than when it remains as part of the whole of a naturally occurring plant organism. In such concentrated form its effect is usually more precise or (to put it another way) more one-sided, and it is usually administered in much higher doses than those initially present in the plant. This frequently produces a toxic effect, which often leads to addiction or habituation, thus reversing the desired healing effect.

We must never forget that human beings on this planet are totally dependent on plants. We have had thousands of years to develop this symbiotic relationship with the plant kingdom. The chemical substances produced by the metabolic processes of plants are very similar to those made by the bodies of humans and animals, and thus our bodies respond to them with few unwanted side effects. By contrast, we have only had a few short decades to accustom ourselves to the products of scientific chemistry and, at best, this situation has produced questionable results.

In the past all medications came directly from nature, with the main source being the plant world. One of the oldest pieces of documentary evidence concerning the use of medicinal herbs is an herbal by the Chinese emperor and physician Shen Nung, in which he set down his knowledge concerning the herbal medicine of that time. The understanding of applying medicinal herbs has developed continuously over thousands of years. Time and again we have asked ourselves how it was that the earliest primal people came to know about herbs. And we have imagined how Neanderthal man, driven by pain and hunger, gradually learned through blind trial and error which plants were edible and which poisonous, which ones had power to heal and which were poisonous, until human beings had at last collected enough practical knowledge to be able to pass it on safely and accurately from generation to generation, right down to the present day.

In fact, the oldest documentary evidence and ethnological research regarding "uncivilized" peoples shows that tribes of ancient times always included wise ones who were able to see behind appearances and perceive the supernatural, spiritual qualities of objects and living things. This special kind of perception applied to people and conditions, and to the nature of plants as well. By disciplined practice and self-induced states of altered consciousness, these wise men and women were able to communicate with plants from the depth of their souls. There is much, in our opinion, to support the belief that these ancients knew more about plants and herbs than we do today.

The beginning of modern times marks a distinct gap in our knowledge of herbs and medicinal plants, for scientific chemistry developed then against the background of industrialization; medicinal herbs were no longer regarded as living entities, but only as isolated chemical structures. In the twentieth century, it even became possible to rearrange the structure of molecules to create completely new, synthetic substances. A new age was born that was going to bless us all with a synthetic solution for every problem we faced in life. Until the nineteenth century, 90 percent of all medicaments were of herbal origin. Less than one hundred years later, the chemical industry has grown into a megapower that offers us sixty thousand plastics, more than fifty thousand artificial herbicides, pesticides, and industrial chemicals, and thirty-thousand synthetic drug medications—all produced entirely in laboratories! The direct damage and the unforeseeable risks that these chemical substances have brought to our lives and our health have only started to become apparent since the 1960s or 1970s.

Academic medicine has developed on the basis of the promises of chemical drugs. The method of treatment is basically symptomatic and finally leads to widespread misuse and overconsumption of medicaments, the long-term consequences of which now seriously threaten the community health of all industrialized countries. Although it has been possible to eradicate innumerable life-threatening diseases and epidemics by means of these powerful drugs, we are no longer able to deceive ourselves that we are in control. Less severe diseases, chronic and functional disorders, and the various autonomic disturbances are on the increase! And what of the new epidemics of our age, cancer and AIDS?

The fundamental disadvantage of chemical drugs lies in their side effects. We have been taught by the medical establishment that we should accept not only the positive effects produced by synthetic drugs but their negative side effects as well. The term "side effect" literally means "to put aside" and this is how the unwanted results become rationalized or trivialized. Yet they are anything but harmless!

In part the renaissance of medicinal herbs is due to the fact that herbs offer solutions without stumbling blocks for everyday disorders. Several recent opinion studies carried out in Europe have revealed people's strong preference for medications of natural origin. No more than 20 percent of those surveyed prefer synthetic chemical preparations because they expect these to be superior in their effect. This changing attitude—

back to nature and away from the blind endorsement of technology that prevailed only a few short years ago—was caused in part by the environmental catastrophes of our recent past (Chernobyl, toxic waste scandals, pollution of rivers and lakes, the extermination of animals and plants). To quote an ancient Chinese sage, "If you do not change your direction, you will undoubtedly end up where you are headed." Thank God the spirit of the times is changing direction.

If we set ourselves at a little distance from our present situation and observe it through the eyes of history, it becomes evident that the return to medicinal herbs and to many ancient methods of natural healing are the necessary response to the extremes of academic medicine. The prediction can also be made that this movement, once it has had time to penetrate the hearts and minds of the people on our planet, will in turn bring about yet another counterreaction. We are convinced that the evolutionary development of medicine and related sciences will lead to ever less crude and careless healing methods, to the use of the energies of more subtle, yet more powerful medications. And perhaps the consciousness of the twenty-first century will lead once again to our rescue from disease, illness, and affliction, through the bounty of healing herbs from God's pharmacy.

❧ 4 ❧

HANDLING AND PREPARING HERBS PROPERLY

One must not only have the knowledge, but also apply it. One must not only desire, but also act.
Johann Wolfgang von Goethe

At the beginning, what really fascinated us most about herbology was the task of collecting the herbs ourselves. In the process you learn to differentiate one herb from another, how to locate the correct variety of a specific species—and much more about the vast world of herbs.

LEARN ABOUT HERBS BY COLLECTING THEM YOURSELF

By collecting herbs yourself, you are compelled to be in close relationship with nature. Every medicinal plant has its typical location, depending on soil type, mineral composition, moisture content, elevation, sunlight, shade, terrain, and so forth. For example, cotton grass, an old traditional cough remedy, grows only in unspoiled virgin moorland. Even in a field that lies immediately next to moorland it would not have the proper living conditions and thus would not thrive at all. The powerful medicinal plant arnica is generally found not at lower altitudes but rather at heights ranging from 2,400 to 7,500 feet; furthermore, it is limited to rough pasture or alpine meadows with lime-free soil. Common club moss, a type of creeping moss, also grows in higher altitudes, but in abundance only beneath the shady boughs of pine trees. As soon as the trees are cut and the ground is directly exposed to sunlight, the club moss disappears.

On the other hand, thyme, that veteran of cold remedies, cannot exist without a great deal of sun. It thrives in dry ground, and the plant loves to cascade over rock walls and bask in the blazing sun. Only under such conditions will it come into flower and exude its heady aroma. Most herbs with a high content of essential oils are sun worshipers; their scent and their medicinal properties do not develop until they are exposed to the radiant warmth of direct and intense sunlight.

Certain herbs have a preference for dry gravel pits, even dumps; these include stinging nettle and the willow-herb. Others are actually partial to being trampled on by people and animals; one such herb is plantain, which grows right alongside well-traveled paths and in meadows and front yards. Another is chicory, which enjoys the sides of dusty streets heavy with traffic.

When you collect herbs yourself, you begin to observe the whole countryside in this new light. Hillocks, hollows, valleys, streams, brooks, woods, slopes, meadows, and forests all speak to you about the herbs living within them. Even when driving along in your car, you can easily recognize which plants will thrive where.

DISCOVERY OF NATURE

To study and experience nature is one of the most beautiful things in life. To be sure, you don't focus on plants to the exclusion of the animals, rocks, and rivers, and the natural beauty surrounding them. When you are outdoors in nature you are constantly provided with new discoveries, things to touch, smell, feel, taste—always something to delight in.

When you collect herbs yourself, you learn about them by experiencing them, by being with them. You experience a plant with all your senses, and as a result, you can intuitively grasp its character, its true nature, and even its purpose. You acquire a feeling for a particular medicinal plant, which is a distinct advantage when studying them more intellectually later on. All this can help you make the right selection of herbs for a certain individual in specific circumstances or put together a well-balanced herbal formula.

Whenever we have led excursions for herbs, we have always endeavored to teach those who came along to open their eyes and see nature surrounding them. Everything that grows needs to be taken in with the eyes, nose, hand, skin, and tongue (which can obviously be dangerous if you don't know what you're doing). It is unfortunate that most people have forgotten how to sense the world around them. In the United States we were particularly surprised at how little people relate to nature. They rarely go for walks in the country, so how can they develop a love of nature? By contrast, Europeans have acquired from their ancestors the habit of going for frequent walks in the woods or fields; even among dyed-in-the-wool city dwellers, hiking is still a very popular activity for young and old alike.

REQUIREMENTS FOR HERB COLLECTING

The beginning herbalist should on no account go about blithely collecting and tasting plants without expert advice! There are many luscious-looking poisonous berries, flowers, and roots, not to mention mushrooms. You must know what you're doing if you want to harvest herbs growing in the wild.

In addition, it is also essential to know which part of the plant possesses healing powers as well as the proper time to harvest herbs. With many medicinal plants all the parts above ground are used (when these are dried the pharmacist refers to them as *herba,* meaning "herb"). *In our formulas throughout the book, whenever we do not specify plant parts such as flowers, leaves, root, and so on, it means that* herba *is used.* With other plants only the flower is harvested (pharmaceutical terminology calls it *flos,* plural *flores*). In both cases the optimal time for collecting is when the plant has just started to bloom. That's when the herb is at the zenith of its vitality, containing all the powers of its inner chemical components and essences which are spent by the time its flower has begun to fade.

Many times we use the leaves of the plant (for which the Latin term is *folia*). In the case of many springtime herbs, which are best eaten as salad or used for flavoring or for blood purification cures—for example, dandelion, stinging nettle, or birch leaves—the fresh tender leaves are picked only when they are pale green and not yet fully mature. At this time they still taste mild and delicate, yet they contain all the essential substances necessary for cleansing and purifying our bodies.

Great care is to be taken when the roots of medicinal plants are to be used (for which the botanical term is *radix*). They must be carefully dug to prevent damage, and a part of the root must remain in the ground so that the plant can continue to live and propagate. The best time for digging roots is in the fall, when the growing power has receded from the flower, stem, and leaves and has returned back into the roots, or in the early spring, when it has yet to move upward to the rest of the plant.

Seeds and fruits are harvested when they are ripe (fruits go under the Latin name *fructus,* seeds under *semen*). If you know the difference between a ripe and unripe pear, for example, with regard to its aroma, taste, and juiciness, you can vividly imagine the difference between ripe and prematurely harvested fennel seeds or rose hips.

Note that it may be important for you to recognize the botanical names and scientific terms associated with plants. When you want to make certain that you are buying or choosing the correct herb, *always go by the Latin name,* because the botanical names are international and standardized, whereas common or folk names of herbs vary even from region to region within the same country, often causing confusion. (Please see the index of herb names in English and Latin.)

PROBLEMS OF HARVESTING WILD HERBS

Apart from all the factors that you must be aware of when gathering plants, collecting medicinal herbs today presents considerable problems, because so many of our known medicinal plants are threatened by extinction. The fact that people have thoughtlessly ripped them out in an uncontrolled manner for many decades has decimated their numbers. As a consequence, many rare herbs, in particular alpine herbs and moorland plants, have come under protection and may no longer be gathered. Of course, one of the main causes of the alarming reduction in species of our flora is something else: the as yet unchecked creep of civilization into the last recesses of unspoiled moorlands, mountain meadows, savannas, marshes, fields, and heaths. The ecological niches of countless plants have consequently been diminished so radically that they no longer have any chance of survival. Sadly, the same applies to the many animals that are completely dependent on interacting with plants for their needs. (We often wonder what will happen to human beings, for we depend on plants and animals as well.)

The most important reason by far for the dramatic restructuring and impoverishment of our plant world, however, is the decades-long use of artificial fertilizers, chemical herbicides, synthetic pesticides, and other so-called plant-protecting agents that are put to work in our food-producing fields. Wherever cultivation involves these synthetic chemicals, medicinal herbs are sure to disappear. No horsetail, chamomile, or cornflowers will grow in these fields. Valerian and cowslip do not thrive in fertilized meadows.

A real and present hazard is posed by our collecting herbs in unsuitable places, those ruined by pesticides and other toxins used in modern agriculture, by the heavy metals generated in streets and highways heavy with traffic, by pollutants in our rivers and streams, and by the airborne plague of acid rain. As a matter of fact, you can now safely collect herbs only in remote areas and high mountain regions; otherwise you do best to purchase your herbs from dealers who can assure you of products free of chemical residue and environmental pollutants.

Today, the majority of medicinal plants used for manufacturing medications are commercially grown, that is, in controlled environments under supervised conditions. This poses a distinct disadvantage for the plant's internal chemical composition, which will be slightly different from that of a similar plant growing wild in nature. On the other hand, a plant grown in a cultivated field under controlled conditions can be protected from many external pollutants, insofar as the cultivation is carried out in a biologically sensible manner. These plants may even be grown in ways that optimize their active ingredients. The controversy as to whether one or another advantage or disadvantage will win out will occupy herbal experts and the pharmaceutical industry for some time to come. Yet not all the medicinal herbs we need can be easily cultivated, for the reasons mentioned before. Some still have to be collected in the wild, just as they have been for thousands of years. Therefore, the profession of herb collector should be a secure one well into the future.

GROWING HERBS IN YOUR OWN GARDEN

Another excellent way to work with herbs is to grow them in your own garden. Of course, this applies to a relatively limited number and variety of plants. Many of them are commonly more familiar as culinary herbs, although they actually possess a medicinal effect. As with many things in life, it is all a matter of viewpoint. If we call a plant a flavoring or cooking herb, then we define it as something that gives our food a certain taste characteristic (for example, caraway seed, parsley, lemon balm, or mint). If we call it a medicinal herb, then we define it as something with healing effect (such as St. Johnswort). If we refer to a plant as a weed, it becomes something undesirable, bothersome, and worthy of being destroyed. If we refer to it as a vegetable, it becomes a plant that is cultivated in order to enrich our diet.

In fact, many herbs are all of these things at the same time; flavoring herb, medicinal herb, weed, and vegetable. A perfect example is the stinging nettle. When dried and ground, stinging nettle leaves lend a delightful tartness to salad dressings. If the entire herb is used to make a tea, it has a diuretic and blood-cleansing effect. Stinging nettle leaves as a vegetable have an excellent taste and stimulate kidney function as well. Gardeners tend to rip it out when it takes over deserted places in the garden. Children hate it when it stings their legs as they romp through meadows in summer. And yet this same stinging, burning sensation was observed generations ago to be helpful as an effective local stimulation therapy for rheumatic pain when the aching joints and muscles are simply touched with the herb. Whenever an herb is suitable for being grown in your own garden it will be mentioned in the following chapters where we describe each herb in detail. Chapter 18 gives detailed instructions for creating your own herb garden.

HOW TO DRY HERBS

Let's suppose you have collected some marvelous, aromatic herbs in an unspoiled, natural area. What do you do with them? Unless you are going to use them fresh, for example in a salad, they must be preserved, which is best done by the process of drying. (Alternative methods of preparation, such as alcohol-water tinctures or extracting fresh plants with oil, will be discussed in later passages.) Drying is a very gentle method of preservation that has been used for thousands of years. Although during the drying process the water will be removed from the herb, the majority of its active ingredients and by-substances will remain present and intact. Drying herbs properly is not all that easy. They must be harvested in a dry state, that is, not when it has been raining or when they are moist with dew. Moreover, they need to be dried in a shady, well-aired location at a temperature not to exceed 105° F. Subjecting herbs to direct sunlight causes them to fade in color and will destroy many or all of their active substances, which is also the reason why they should be stored after drying in tinted jars protected from the light.

Herbs dry best when they are loosely spread on a cotton or linen sheet stretched over a wooden grate and turned over at least every other day. This method is preferable to tying them in bunches and hanging them up, as the latter method causes the stems and leaves to become somewhat crushed, and they tend to dry more slowly and unevenly, are apt to mildew, and acquire an unappealing appearance.

HOW TO STORE DRIED HERBS

When the herb is so dry that it rustles and crumbles easily to the touch, break it up by hand or with a knife or scissors so that the pieces can easily go into a storage jar. The average piece should be approximately three-quarters of an inch in length. Stems sometimes become quite hard and must be cut up into smaller pieces—a tedious task. Delicate flower petals, of course, will dry more quickly than pulpy leaves, fruits, or roots. For work with roots we recommend the use of a drying cabinet or kiln, as the drying process otherwise takes many weeks and the danger of mildew is far greater.

As a rule, dried herbs should not be kept longer than about two years. We refer to dried herbs as being "fresh" for this entire time. (For those who can harvest herbs themselves, one year is the preferred maximum). If the supply of herbs has not been used up by then, they can always be used for external applications such as herbal baths. Dried herbs must be stored in clean, dry receptacles and be kept as air-tight as possible. Ceramic, wood, tin, or (preferably) glass jars and containers are suitable. Lined paper bags that seal in the aroma, similar to the bags used for coffee or tea, are also acceptable for short-term storage so long as they are tightly sealed.

When working with herbs you have gathered yourself, *always remember to carefully label each container* with the name of the herb or herb mixture and the date on which they were stored. *This is a must!*

For a pharmacist, proper labelling is a cardinal rule, and if you wish in any sense to become your own pharmacist, it is best to act like one.

Taking into consideration the expense, time, work, and space requirements, as well as the experience needed to grow, collect, dry, and store your own herbs, it may not be worth all the effort required. Still, it is both fun and educational, and you should certainly try it for the sheer experience and enjoyment involved. But collecting herbs is not necessary if you are basically interested in knowing how to apply herbs correctly. Many fine herb stores carry a wonderful selection of fresh herbs and herbal preparations for you to use instead. (See also "Herbal Suppliers," page 269.)

TYPES OF HERBAL PREPARATIONS

Although *herbal tea* is certainly the best-known preparation method, it is by no means the only one or even the best one in every case. There are a number of possibilities, and your success depends on choosing the best one appropriate for each unique situation, as we will explain in the following chapters. Many herbs are most effective as a *tincture* (in the form of an alcohol extract; an example is shepherd's purse). Some herbs develop their greatest effect as an *herbal bath* or when used by *inhalation*, especially those which contain a lot of essential oils (such as thyme). Others are best suited for external or topical use, in the form of an *ointment* (such as calendula). Certain herbs (arnica, for example) are hazardous when administered orally, yet when used externally have a wonderful curative effect. Some herbs, herbal preparations, or mixtures are most effective when applied as a *moist dressing* or *compress* (example: Swedish Bitters), while others are best applied as a *dry compress* (example: chamomile flowers). Various herbs are at their most powerful when they are consumed in the form of *fresh-squeezed juice, salad, or fresh vegetable* (stinging nettle, for instance). Occasionally the same plant will show a variety of different effects depending on how it is extracted, that is, with water as a tea, with alcohol as a tincture, or with vegetable oil (example: St. Johnswort). All these methods of preparation have proved themselves in the rich tradition of medicinal herbs that extends back for thousands of years. To associate herbs merely with tea is only scratching the surface.

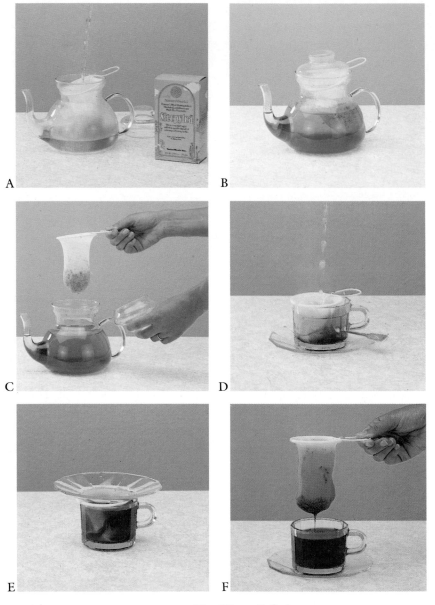

FIGURE 1. *Hot Water Infusion*

A. Place herbs in tea net, hang tea net over the teapot, and pour boiling water over the net to cover the herbs.

B. Cover the teapot and allow the herbs to steep.

C. When the steeping time is up, remove the tea net containing the herbs.

D. For one cup of tea, place one to two teaspoonsful of herbs in a tea net, hang the net over the cup, and pour boiling water over it.

E. Cover the cup and allow to steep.

F. When the steeping time is up, remove the tea net.

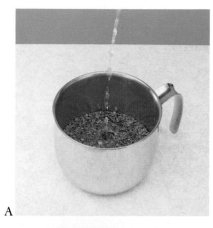

A

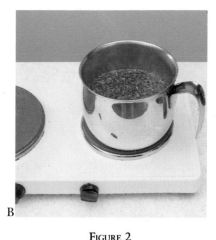

B

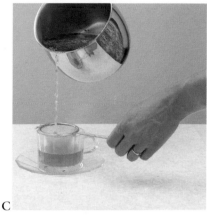

C

FIGURE 2

Cold Water Infusion

A. Place herbs in a pot, cover with cold water, and allow to steep overnight.
B. In the morning, heat the infusion slightly.
C. Strain off the herbs before use.

The Herbal Tea

To begin with, let's discuss the basic rules for making herbal tea. From the point of view of pharmacology, tea is an aqueous extract of plant parts, with the active ingredients dissolved in water in very minute quantities. When you pour hot boiling water over your herbs to prepare tea, the pharmacist calls such an extract a *hot water infusion* (see figure 1). Sometimes cold water is used instead, so that the herbs are soaked for several hours or overnight and then heated or boiled. This is called a *cold water infusion* (see figure 2). With some herbs it is necessary to extract them in this manner without the use of great heat to protect certain substances (such as the delicate mucins in mallow). Roots, bark, and wood pieces in general must be extracted by first soaking them in cold water, then bringing them to a boil and simmering for between three and ten minutes. The latter method of extraction is called a *decoction*.

Throughout the book the description of each herb or formula will include a discussion of how best to prepare it. If no specific direction is given, you will always know to use the simple hot water infusion.

Extraction Time

With respect to the method of extraction, it is possible to make a tea from either fresh or dried herbs. The cardinal rule is that the thinner and softer the plant parts being used, the shorter the extraction time; the harder and more impenetrable the plant, the longer the extraction time and/or the higher the temperature. For example, in order to prepare an elder flower tea with a delicious aroma, boiling water is simply poured over the fresh or dried flowers and the mixture is allowed to steep for about three minutes. In order to effectively extract a kidney-bladder tea containing relatively hard constituents, such as horsetail and juniper berries, the mixture must be allowed to steep for as long as ten minutes. To make a strong tea from whole rose hips, you will have to leave it in a kettle at a rolling boil for ten minutes, as the kernels are extremely hard. Extraction in this case is intensified by increased temperature and longer extraction time. To prepare an effective liver-gallbladder tea consisting for the most part of bitter roots such as angelica and chicory, the herb and water mixture must be allowed to soak overnight and then brought to a boil for a moment in the morning. In this example, the duration of the extraction is increased. In ready-mixed teas, harder and softer plant parts are combined, so that an average extraction time of about five minutes is in order.

Another cardinal rule is that the tea pot or cup be covered with a lid (or saucer) while the tea is steeping or brewing. Essential oils and other active ingredients are extremely volatile (that is, apt to escape into the air) and need to be contained in this manner. They also collect in drops of condensation on the underside of the lid and should be returned to the extract by shaking them back in.

The Cotton Tea Bag

The simplest and, we feel, best device for making tea is a cotton tea bag or tea net that hangs from a wire down into the cup or tea pot and can be gently swayed back and forth. This way the tea does not need to be strained through a sieve when the extraction is completed; the particles are removed by the cotton bag and stay within it to be disposed of later.

Cotton tea nets can be purchased at natural food stores (see "Herbal Suppliers," page 269). Even with daily use they will last for about one year. We do not recommend using a "tea ball," because the herbs are packed too tightly inside the ball and are not sufficiently flushed through when the particles are soaked in water and expand in size. Not only is the coloring of tea important, but even more vital is that the major active ingredients are dissolved. Tea with a dark coloring may indicate that many substances have been dissolved out of the herbs—but they may not necessarily be those that are of importance in connection with a certain therapy.

Quantities

The rule of thumb when making herbal tea is one to two heaping teaspoonsful of dried herb to one cup water, depending upon your past experience with the herb and how strong you want the tea. This measure is relatively accurate for store-bought herbs, because they are normally cut to a standard size, although seeds and flowers, for example, are quite different in size and shape.

When it comes to fresh-picked herbs, it is difficult to give precise quantities because of the wide variations in size, weight, and structure of different plant parts. When using fresh-picked herbs, the rule of thumb is to use three times the quantity you would use of dried herb. The extraction time is much shorter with fresh-picked herbs because they are much softer and thus are quickly penetrated by the water. For example, in making a tea from fresh stinging nettle leaves, only one to two minutes of steeping time is required, whereas three to five minutes are needed to steep the dried leaves.

Since it is so difficult to give any hard and fast rules for the quantities required for making tea from fresh-picked herbs, we recommend that you experiment for yourself. This is the wisest course, all the more so because it is ultimately your sense of taste that will be the determining factor. Obviously, the majority of herb users will rely on store-bought herbs, but we do encourage you to try fresh-picked herbs when the time of year and the time in your life permit you to enjoy them.

Finally, please note that in this revised edition, we have given all formulas in parts rather than in grams, as was the case in the first edition. Although professional herbalists and pharmacists in the United States and worldwide can easily cope with grams because they are used to working with the established international measuring system, the feedback from our American readers has been that they encounter numerous problems with the metric system in their private households. Not only did our readers find it very difficult to measure such minute quantities as 2, 3, or 5 grams, household scales with gram measurements are hard to obtain in the United States.

On the other hand, if we had given the formulas in ounces, our Canadian, African, Asian, and English-speaking readers around the world would have been discriminated against. So the best solution to satisfy all needs seemed to be the simplification into parts. For us, the authors, it meant reformulating a few of the recipes and accepting the disadvantage of being less precise. Less precise we are now because it makes a difference whether you measure herbs by volume (parts, teaspoons, etc.), or by weight (grams or ounces); e.g., a tablespoon of balm leaves weighs 3 grams, a tablespoons of rose hips weighs 9 grams. Nevertheless, we made sure that this change will not cause the formulas to be any less effective or safe. As always, our first and foremost goal with this book is to be practical.

Your own needs will tell you what to use as one part: a teaspoon, a tablespoon, a small yogurt cup, or a mug. When you buy a ready-made tea mixture, you'll generally find it packed in 80 or 100 grams, or 3 to 4 ounces; tinctures range from 30 to 100 grams, or 1 to 4 ounces.

This is a good amount for short-term therapy. Here and there we have also recommended simple teas consisting of one, two, or three herbs. In such cases a formula is not needed. Simply mix equal parts of each different herb to prepare the tea. As you gain more experience, you may want to adjust the quantities of one or another herb to create your own special mixture.

Improving the Taste of Your Teas

Even when a medicinal effect should take priority, we endeavor to give our teas as pleasant a taste as possible. After all, what good is a tea that is quite effective but tastes so bad you can't bring yourself to drink it? In a liver-gallbladder tea, for example, the many components that contain bitter substances have to be balanced by pleasant-tasting, less specifically acting herbs such as blackberry and raspberry leaves. In the herbal industry even the appearance of the tea mixture is important, which is why one often adds a dash of yellow calendula flowers and blue cornflowers to give it a little color. This requires creative ability as well as experience, characteristics much like those of an accomplished cook.

All teas may be sweetened as desired, with the exception of those mixtures where we mention specifically not to do so. Being health-conscious, we avoid sugar and use honey, maple or grain syrup, or concentrated fruit juice instead. Often, a small touch of freshly squeezed orange or lemon gives the tea mixture a final and delightful touch. We should do everything possible to make our daily medicine as pleasurable as possible.

The Importance of Water

Water plays a triple role in making tea. First, it is the extraction medium. Second, it is the vehicle or carrier of the dissolved chemical ingredients. Third, it functions in the body as a flushing agent. The intestinal villi can assimilate the tea mixture along with its medicinal agents very easily and quickly, even when an individual is unable to eat any solid foods. In addition, natural-health practitioners recommend drinking at least two to three quarts of liquid each day to assure that the digestive juices and tissue fluids are continually irrigated. The optimal way of taking specifically medicinal teas is to sip the hot or warm tea about every fifteen minutes throughout the day. In this way, the body is subtly stimulated to react and is thus allowed to compensate for the health disturbance itself. For the sake of practicality, we recommend that a sufficient quantity of tea be made each morning and kept close by in a thermos bottle during the day.

MIXING HERBS

Because every medicinal herb has a different composition and structure, it is useful to combine various kinds of herbs into tea mixtures. This enables the herbs to work synergistically and thus to act on certain functional disturbances from a variety of different angles. A classic cough tea, for example, will contain all sorts of herbs that act on the lungs, bronchial tubes, and mucous membranes; however, one component has a soothing effect, another a mucolytic (mucus-dissolving) action, a third is an expectorant, and a fourth a disinfecting agent, while the fifth ingredient generally replenishes the body's natural defense mechanisms. Herein lies the true essence of the art of the herbalist or herbal pharmacist: in creating the optimal formula or recipe.

In general, we have achieved best results with dried, loose bulk herbs, since they are the most natural. However, in certain situations it may be a great help to have an instant herbal tea. Such a tea is prepared by simply adding either hot or cold water to the instant tea powder. For a long time we resisted recommending any such instant tea, because they all were produced using a base made from white sugar. Recently, however, a pure protein base has been developed in Germany on which the herb extract can be sprayed. Since this protein base is completely water soluble and tasteless and contains next to no calories, such a tea is very appropriate for diabetic patients and others who wish to avoid sugar. Of course these instant teas are very convenient for people on the go, since all that is needed to prepare the tea is a little water. It need not even be hot water: cold water will do the job just as well.

For the sake of completeness, we also want to mention that we do not think it is the best thing to swallow pulverized herbs in capsules. Not only are many natural ingredients destroyed in the process of pulverization, but also the body is often unable to assimilate the respective chemical ingredients from the herb powder without their being extracted in some medium first.

HERBAL BATHS

In many cases, an herbal bath is a very effective application. It can be used as a full bath or a partial body bath, such as a sitz bath or footbath. The preparation of the herbs is almost exactly the same as for a tea, only that you use much larger quantities of herbs and water and in general prepare a very strong extract. Depending on the size of your bathtub or container, you use one to three handfuls of herb with one to three quarts of water. When the extraction is completed (by letting the herbs soak overnight and/or bringing them slowly to a boil), the herbs must be strained through a large kitchen sieve and then poured into the tub (see figure 3). Take heed not to burn yourself! Whenever we recommend such a treatment we indicate the larger quantities and the best method of extraction. Complete the preparation by diluting the herb infusion with water added at body temperature.

Sitz baths have proved to be most helpful, not only in many cases of abdominal spasms and cramps but also for chronic kidney infections, vaginal infections, and the like. The best results here are achieved with a special sitz-bath tub where only your lower abdomen and lower back rest in the warm or hot water, while your upper body from the waist up plus your legs and feet are out of the water. If you don't have such a special container, you can take a sitz bath in a regular bathtub by simply sitting in it instead of lying down.

Specific external applications like douches and washings of certain body parts are also prepared in the same way. The difference is again that we need smaller quantities of herbs and water and different containers as well.

Herbal inhalations are also prepared as simple infusions. (Please see the illustrations on page 77.) Here it is important to have everything at hand before you begin and to act quickly, because it is the volatile essential oils that promote healing in this case, and these simply evaporate if you wait ten minutes before actually inhaling them.

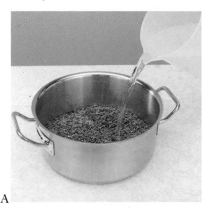

A

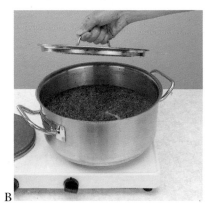

B

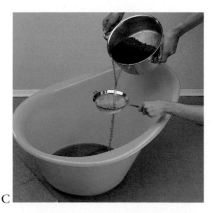

C

FIGURE 3.   *Herbal Bath*

(The illustration shows the preparation of a horsetail sitz bath.)

A. Steep herbs in cold water for several hours or overnight.
B. Place the pot on a stove, heat slowly to a boil, cover, and allow to steep again.
C. Strain off the herbs, pour the decoction into bathtub or sitz bath container, and add warm water (for a sitz bath, enough water to reach the lower back).

HERBAL TINCTURES

Herbal tinctures are alcoholic extractions of either fresh or dried herbs with an alcohol content varying from 80 to 140 proof, depending on the plant material being extracted. In general a thorough extraction is completed after ten days. Tinctures can be applied both internally and externally and can either enhance or replace treatments with tea—for example, when a very strong and fast effect is needed, or when the patient is traveling and the making of tea is difficult or out of the question. Because tinctures are taken as drops you can administer them very accurately. Tinctures can be stored for a much longer time than dried herbs and will not deteriorate, since the alcohol keeps them fresh and useful for a number of years.

In addition, high-quality tinctures are always "standardized." This means that individual herb substances—active ingredients, aroma substances, trace elements, essential oils, and so on—contained in the tincture are the same from one bottle to the next and, as is the case in Germany, must adhere to strict requirements. The manufacturer of such tinctures can compensate for the natural differences in herbs grown from one area to another or from one growing season to the next by adjusting the extraction procedure to meet a measurable standard. This is most important with regard to the herbs' active ingredients.

For internal use, tinctures can be diluted with herbal tea, water, or juice, or can be dropped directly on the tongue. For external use, the tincture is applied directly to the skin or in the form of poultices.

Herbal Tinctures and Homeopathic Tinctures

People are often confused about the difference between *herbal tinctures* and *homeopathic tinctures*. These two categories are quite different, not only in the general idea of their application but also in the specific method of their preparation. The regular herbal tincture in phytotherapy is made from dried herbs with one part herb to ten parts alcohol/water. The homeopathic tincture is prepared from fresh herbs only by extracting one part herb to one or two parts alcohol/water. This basic tincture is called the "mother tincture" and is further diluted in a ratio of 1:10 (i.e., one part mother tincture plus nine parts alcohol/water): the resulting mixture is referred to as 2x. A 3x mixture is one part of the 2x mixture diluted with nine more parts alcohol/water, and so on. Each time a homeopathic dilution is made the mixture is succussed, that is, vigorously shaken a specified number of times.

Ever since its invention by the German physician Samuel Hahnemann (1755–1843), homeopathy has been the subject of great controversy. Those who are used to dealing with material substances hold that a dilution above 23x (1 x 10^{-23}) does not contain even a single molecule of the active ingredient of the herb. Hence, they assert, it cannot work. Yet those who conceive of plants and plant extracts as being more than an arrangement of active and ancillary "material" substances—in other words, who view them as rich informational energy-patterns as well—work very effectively with these homeopathic preparations, especially with the higher potencies (10x, 15x, 100x, etc.).

We think that with our increasing ability to define and measure even the minutest quantities and actions of chemical substances by the use of highly sensitive and sophisticated instruments, it no longer seems a mystery that effects can be brought about by these subtle vibrational energies. Perhaps proof of this is the action of hormones within our bodies. These highly effective physiological substances direct all our organs, yet they exist only in the most minute quantities. For example, the hormones of the pituitary gland (hypophysis) still work in quantities of one millesimal (thousandth) of a milligram. Adrenalin, the hormone produced by the suprarenal glands, acts the same even in dilution ratios as small as 1:1,000,000,000,000 (one to one trillion)!

Although herbology and homeopathy often use the same herbs to begin with, they sometimes differ in their indications (fields of application) because of each method's differing interpretation of symptoms and way of diagnosing—in short, the two directions espouse entirely distinct systems of treatment. In homeopathy even highly poisonous plant, animal, or mineral substances can be taken internally. Because of the high dilutions, they obviously cannot do any harm but rather act as medicinal agents. Phytotherapy works with cruder substances and higher dosages of chemical ingredients. It also isn't as complicated a system to learn as classical homeopathy.

Why Alcohol?

To complete the discussion of herbal tinctures we would like to add some information concerning the use of alcohol in natural medications.

For centuries alcohol has been considered to be an optimal medium for preparing plant medications. From the point of view of the pharmaceutical chemist, not only is alcohol indispensable for extracting the active ingredients, it is also required to stabilize and preserve them. For alcohol has the ability to inhibit enzymatic or hydrolytic reactions in plant extracts as well as to limit microbe activity.

In addition to its function as a solvent and preservative, alcohol also plays a role as a carrier substance for conveying active ingredients within the body. It has been scientifically proved that alcohol increases the permeability of the mucous coat of the stomach. Alcohol promotes the resorption of small quantities of chemically unstable plant ingredients by way of a variety of mechanisms in the intestinal wall. In certain conditions, alcohol additionally supplements and promotes the healing effect on the target organs.

Furthermore, it has been scientifically established that minute quantities of alcohol do improve the resistance of the immune defense system (reticulo-endothelial system) and are also, surprisingly, able to protect against the threat of coronary arteriosclerosis and heart attack. Comprehensive epidemiological studies show that a higher percentage of teetotalers die of heart attack than other individuals and that a quantity of alcohol amounting from 1 g to a maximum of 40 g per day considerably reduces the risk of heart attack. This corresponds to an average of one glass of wine per day. This should come as a welcome relief to some, for in this day of more and more concern about alcohol consumption it's nice to know there is scientific evidence to suggest that enjoying a glass of your favorite wine may be good for your health. In any event, the dose of alcohol contained in medications such as those we describe never exceeds 4 g to 8 g per day (tinctures being administered by the drop and tonics by the teaspoon), whereas according to recent studies, the danger of liver damage does not arise unless daily quantities of 140 g for women and 210 g for men are consumed for years on end. Finally, for those who want to or who must avoid alcohol completely, it will be helpful to know that when drops of tincture are added to hot water or hot tea the alcohol evaporates immediately.

Other specific preparations of herbs, such as oil extractions or other applications (e.g., wet or dry compresses) are explained in detail elsewhere whenever we recommend such treatments.

❧ 5 ❧

YOUR FIRST STEP: CLEANSING

People pray to the gods for health, yet it is in their own hands to keep it. They do not consider that by their excesses they create the contrary and by their unchecked desires they betray their own health.

Democritus

According to Dr. Otto Buchinger, the German naturopath pioneer of healing through fasting, fasting is "the royal way to healing." According to another nature-cure physician, Dr. Xaver Meier, "Every illness begins in the intestine." Both comments reflect the traditional wisdom that our health is fundamentally dependent upon what we eat, the soundness of our digestive system, and the vitality of our inner metabolic processes—in other words, upon our degree of "purity." In the United States, outstanding success has been achieved with colonics (flushing of the intestinal tract), a method that has gained widespread popularity over the past ten to fifteen years. In the colonic treatment, a device is used that flushes out the entire large intestine in a fashion similar to an enema, gradually cleaning out all the lodged, hardened bits of food and fecal residue. Not only do people experience the subjective feeling of relief and lightness after such a treatment; objectively verifiable results also clearly demonstrate the usefulness of such cleansing by showing dramatic improvements with regard to allergies, headache, rheumatic pain, neurasthenic conditions, and so forth.

41

FASTING CURES

It is a blessing that a variety of fasting cures have become popular again. They range from casual one-day regimens, through five-day programs for losing weight, to healing fasts lasting as long as three to four weeks. In each case, no solid food is eaten and only fruit or vegetable juices, or herbal teas in particular, are consumed. In numerous fasting clinics it has been observed that such varying complaints as high or low blood pressure, migraine, hemorrhoids, irregular menstrual cycles, acne, depression, and chronic rheumatoid arthritis actually disappear "all by themselves," when the body has the opportunity to be rid of all sorts of toxins and unwanted deposits. As a rule, the body's general defense mechanisms are improved after a fasting cure, so that the physiological regulatory systems can once again take control of the body.

Anyone who has gone through a radical fasting cure knows the astounding extent to which our emotions and our thought processes are determined by what we eat and drink and by the impurities circulating in our blood. That person also knows the feeling of relief and lightness, clarity, serenity, refreshment, and brightness one can have on completing such a cleansing. There is no better way of experiencing just how deeply interrelated is the well-being of body, mind, and soul.

The fasting cure with which we have achieved excellent results is based on the experiences of Dr. Buchinger and was described by Dr. Hellmut Lützner. We begin with a radical evacuation of the intestinal tract by using a purgative salt, and then drink only liquids for the next ten to sixteen days. We drink one cup of warm vegetable broth and one glass of fresh juice each day, and otherwise many cups of herbal tea. Since one tends to feel cold because of a somewhat lowered rate of blood circulation during fasting, the hot or warm tea is always a delight, even in summer. Our daily schedule of activities includes plenty of exercise and yoga practice, swimming, walking, hiking, or jogging interspersed with resting periods, a liver compress, and an enema every day. We always take time off from work for this rejuvenating cure, because we want to dedicate our attention fully to this process of inner and outer, physical and spiritual recharging.

During fasting cures, evacuative and blood-purifying tea mixtures are especially advisable, as are those that more specifically stimulate the liver, the kidneys, and/or the circulatory system. In this way, minor crises that occur during fasting can be overcome and the efficiency of the cure greatly improved. Of course, even if you are not fasting you can enjoy some of the benefits of blood-cleansing herbs. You can use them when on a normal diet or during times when you are on a more simple diet consisting primarily of raw vegetables.

THE SPRING CLEANSING CURE

The time-honored *spring cure* is of major importance in the traditional of herbology. In the old days, when people were closer to nature and its rhythms, the great majority of people farmed the land from spring to fall and lived lives filled with demanding physical labor. Winter was a time of contemplation and physical inactivity with a natural tendency toward rest. As soon as spring was in the air, people became busy and active again. The body had to be prepared for this dramatic change. After a winter of root vegetables and the (by then boring) "put up" foodstuffs, the first tender shoots of herbs and wild-growing vegetables were gathered and eaten with delight and joy. Their metabolism-stimulating effect was amplified by the perspiration of hard work as well as by sauna and steam baths.

The lifestyle of modern people, by contrast, is hardly sensitive to nature's rhythms. Executives, secretaries, and accountants sit in their offices winter and spring, thermostats set constantly at 72° F (22° C), suffering from the effects of too little exercise. Workers always begin their day at the same time, regardless of whether the sun sets early or late that day. Yet our autonomic nervous system is still reacting to changes in weather and season. During these periods of change, we are more sensitive and susceptible to colds. Thus we should give our system all the help we can to enable it to adapt to the new season.

STINGING NETTLE

In our opinion the most powerful blood-purifying herb is stinging nettle (*Urtica dioica*). It drives toxins and metabolic waste products out of the body by stimulating the kidneys to excrete more water. In addition, tea made of fresh or dried stinging nettle also cleanses out the entire intestinal tract and activates the body's natural defense mechanisms. We recommend it as a long-term stimulation therapy for allergies, for per-

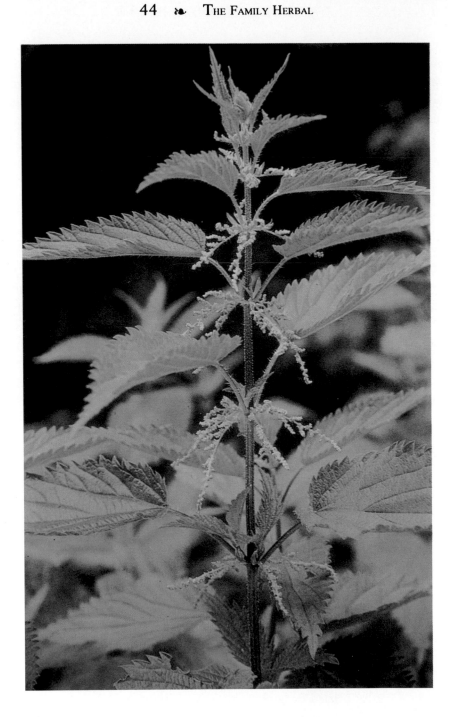

STINGING NETTLE *Urtica dioica*

sons with troubled complexion, and as an additional discharging therapy in connection with all types of rheumatoid diseases and gout. We know of several cases in which hay fever has been completely cured by drinking stinging nettle tea every day from November through April, until the pollen season begins. You can easily observe for yourself that stinging nettle has a diuretic effect: you will urinate more frequently, and in addition the urine will tend to take on a darker color and stronger smell during the first few days of drinking the tea. People who have a predisposition to kidney stones have a chance to prevent them by drinking this tea regularly (see also page 190). The diuretic effect of the stinging nettle is also reflected in the strong urinelike scent of the fully mature plant.

Using Stinging Nettle as a Vegetable

A marvelous gift to your body is a dish of tender stinging nettle leaves, eaten as a vegetable in the spring. At this time of year they do not as yet create the typical burning sensation that is felt when the leaves are touched, and they can be sautéed with onion in oil or butter, much as you would prepare fresh spinach; you should finish up the dish with a bit of cream. This meal, served with potatoes, not only tastes fantastic but has a beneficial effect as well. However, be careful not to overdo it. We know a young man who, in his unbounded enthusiasm for the stinging nettle spring cure, ate it as a vegetable for five days in a row and ended up with an uncomfortable renal colic—a clear-cut case of an overdose! Stinging nettle vegetable should not be eaten more than once a week, and then only in spring so long as the tender, young leaves possess a delicate taste.

Stinging Nettle Tea

Stinging nettle tea has a milder effect than the fresh plant, which is why it can be consumed on a daily basis over six months without causing any harm—insofar as this is not used to flush out edema (water retention) caused by heart or kidney deficiency. However, you should not overdo with this tea either. *Do not drink more than three cups of stinging nettle tea per day.*

A customer came to our pharmacy one day with a terrible skin condition on her face and all over her body. When we asked her what kind of medications she had been using, she proudly answered, "Nothing but stinging nettle tea." When we asked her how much she drank every day, she said, "Three liters" (in other words, more than three quarts). Obviously the inner cleansing process had been initiated too radically and much too abruptly by this overdose. Although we certainly want the body to discharge and the metabolism to be stimulated, we do not want this to happen in such an uncontrolled way, but rather slowly and gently, bit by bit.

Stinging nettle also contains a high amount of iron and therefore promotes the formation of healthy red blood cells. Combined with Swedish Bitters elixir (see chapter 8), stinging nettle makes a highly effective tea to flush from the body low doses of highly toxic substances of every type, especially those which come into our food as the result of pollution.

External Use of Stinging Nettle Tea

Several special external applications can be made using stinging nettle. For example, a hair tonic can be prepared using a diluted tincture made from the plant's roots that will stimulate the circulation in the scalp and eliminate dandruff as well. Furthermore, treating aching muscles and joints as well as muscle tensions by whipping them with a bunch of stinging nettles is surprisingly effective. Along with the skin irritation caused by stinging nettle, the blood circulation is increased in the tissues, and possible deposits or inflammatory processes which cause pain are eliminated from the inside out. Such therapy is certainly not everyone's cup of tea, but in naturopathy, it belongs to the holistic approach whereby well-dosed stimuli are used to force the body to bring forth certain reactions or metabolic changes.

DANDELION

Dandelion (*Taraxacum officinale*) has a purifying effect that is virtually as powerful as that of stinging nettle. It too is one of the spring herbs whose healing power is best utilized by eating it fresh in April and May. Before the trees come into bloom, the meadows are covered with its bright yellow flowers. The sight of these fields sprinkled with yellow is overwhelming, especially in the seemingly endless pasturelands of Bavaria. The habit of eating young, tender dandelion shoots as a salad comes from France, where gourmets have always relished the unique and deli-

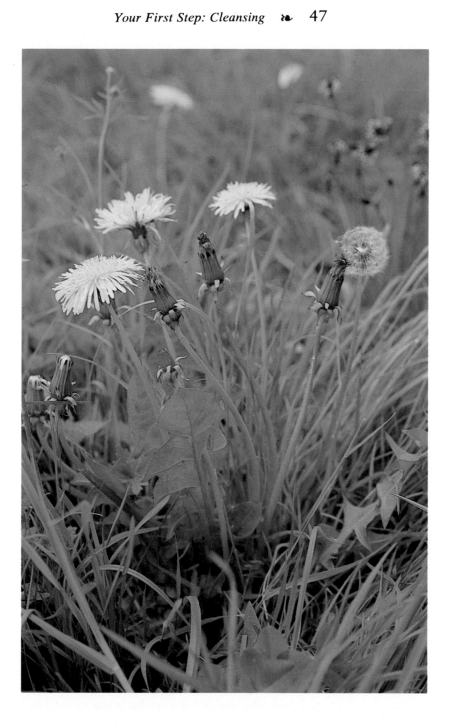

DANDELION *Taraxacum officinale*

cately bitter taste of this wild-growing spring salad favorite. The French were well acquainted with dandelion's diuretic effects; hence its humorous common name *pisse-en-lit*. (In the dialect of our home state Saarland, which borders on France, dandelion is similarly known as *Bettseicher,* or "bed wetter.") Nowadays, two kinds of dandelion are cultivated and available at certain food markets. However, the wild variety has a more powerful and bitter taste.

According to folk belief, the stems and flowers of the dandelion are poisonous. This is not true, but the misconception may be explained by the fact that the stem and leaves when torn exude a sticky white juice that leaves brown stains on hands and clothing. In reality, all parts of the dandelion plant, the leaves, stem, flower, and root, possess healing powers and are easily digestible.

Benefits of Dandelion

Highly valued as a medicinal plant in ancient times, dandelion is described in detail in herb books of the Middle Ages under the name *Herba urinaria*. In addition to the plant's diuretic effect, it is also a wonderful remedy for digestive problems relating to the stomach and the intestines, such as a bloated feeling and the formation of gas. Some herbal experts attribute to dandelion a special effect on the pancreas.

It has been demonstrated that dandelion stimulates the production of bile and eliminates problems relating to proper bile flow. In the chapter on Swedish Bitters (chapter 8), we explain how all bitter substances stimulate the liver. Dandelion is a perfect example of this, as it contains predominantly bitter substances. The liver plays a key role in the purification processes of our bodies. It decides which substances are to be excreted, which are to be stored, transformed, or created. You should pay special attention to the liver on a fasting cure, as it is the liver's job during a fast to clean out the "junk" in all the neglected parts of the organism. By drinking a tea made of dandelion leaves and roots we can support the liver in its monumental job. Unfortunately, this tea does not taste very pleasant to most people; therefore we recommend buffering it with other herbs to create a blood-purifying or liver/gall-stimulating tea mixture (see pages 55 and 165). Dandelion generally has a stimulating and altering effect on the metabolism, which is why it is also used today as a supportive therapy for sciatic neuralgia (excruciating pain in the lower back), lumbago, arthritis, and rheumatism (see page 191).

HORSETAIL

The third plant in the alliance of the great blood purifiers is horsetail (*Equisetum arvense*). It is also referred to as scouring rush, since some species are used as polishing tools because of their abrasive stems. Other names for horsetail are cattail and toadpipe, designations that derive from the appearance of the lacy, bushy plant. As a matter of fact, there are mainly two types of horsetail. *Equisetum arvense,* which grows in crop fields, has healing powers, while *Equisetum palustre,* a taller plant that grows mainly in swamps and wetlands, is poisonous. *It is extremely important that you be able to correctly identify the different varieties.*

Horsetail's Unique Structure

Horsetail is an ancient resident of our planet. Like mosses and ferns, it reproduces asexually by way of spores. It is well worth taking the time to closely examine this plant with your eyes and fingers; you will immediately discover its severe simplicity and rigid structure. Horsetail contains more minerals than most other plants and is very rich in silica, a substance that the body needs to build healthy bones, cartilage, hair, and fingernails. In the form of silicic acid, silica is also indispensable for the healthy condition of the skin and for healing sores and wounds. Regarding its importance for the connective tissue in general and the problem of varicose veins in particular, please see page 228. The jointed stems and leaves of the plant are composed of a series of short shafts successively growing out of one another in telescoping fashion, each of which is connected by a joint and tendonlike sheath. The leaf is reduced to the middle vein and thus resembles the needle of a conifer.

Horsetail's Healing Properties

The plant's hard and stiff quality represents a remarkable parallel to the primary structural element within the human body: the skeleton. The horsetail plant is also a reflection of the spinal column, with its many small pieces of bone connected in jointed fashion, and of joints in general. It should hardly come as a surprise that this medicinal plant also acts on those organs that are most closely associated with the skeletal system—the kidneys. Whenever and wherever joints and bones are weak and degenerative processes are in progress, the cause is sure to be related to an energy deficiency of the kidneys. Weak kidneys are psycho-

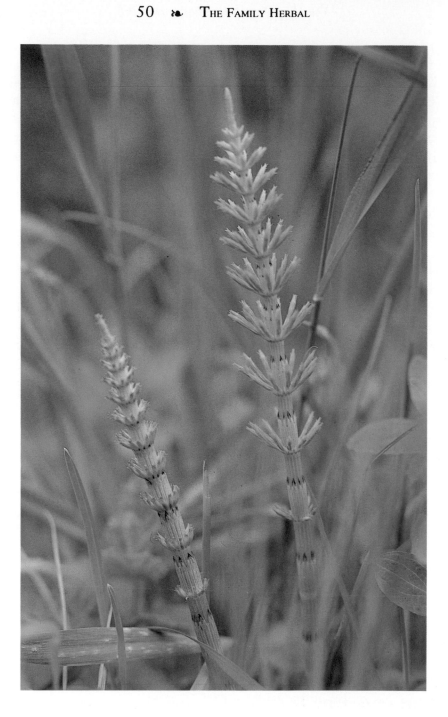

HORSETAIL   *Equisetum arvense*

logically associated with fear, which is why feeling fear makes "your bones go weak" or makes us "weak in the knees." For this reason chronic complaints or disorders of the locomotive apparatus (bones, joints, and related structures), such as rheumatism, gout, and arthrosis, should be treated with medicinal plants that are kidney-activating and diuretic, despite the latest theory from the medical establishment (that these disorders must be attributed to autoimmunization processes and metabolic malfunction).

Horsetail tea is ideal for flushing out the system in connection with bacterial and inflammatory illnesses of the kidneys and urinary tract, as well as renal gravel. (See Chapter 13.) It is also suitable for countering edema (water retention), for example, as a result of traumatic injuries, always with the exception that it not be used for edema that has been caused by impaired cardiac or renal function.

Horsetail Sitz Bath

The beneficial effect of horsetail tea upon inflamed kidneys or kidneys easily susceptible to infections can be considerably enhanced by taking a horsetail sitz bath twice a week. (See pages 37 and 187–188.)

Compresses, Washes, and Baths with Horsetail

Horsetail decoction is also externally administered to support the treatment of slow-healing sores and wounds. Excellent results have also been obtained with baths, washes, or compresses for treating skin diseases that cover large areas, eczema, and festering sores on feet or legs—something from which elderly people often suffer. Such an application begins with the preparation of a horsetail decoction. For a compress use three tablespoonsful of dried herb steeped in a quart of water. For a bath for wounds or for washing wounds, use one and a half handfuls of root and two to three quarts of water. The herb is boiled with the water for ten minutes and then strained out. The foot or leg is bathed in this medium at body temperature; for other parts of the body where this is not possible, hold the wound over an empty bowl or large container and pour the decoction slowly over the afflicted area (see figure 4). If such washing is painful, soak a piece of cotton in the decoction, apply it over the wound, cover it with a dry towel, and make it secure with a bandage or scarf. You can renew this compress again after about half an hour. Afterward, coat the wound (particularly the edges) with calendula oint-

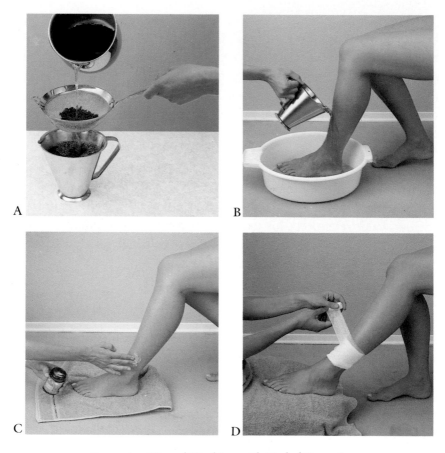

FIGURE 4. *Wound Washing with Herbal Decoction*

A. When the steeping time is up, strain off the herbs and allow the decoction or infusion
    to cool to body temperature.
B. Pour the decoction very slowly over the afflicted area.
C. Apply calendula ointment to the wound and its edges.
D. Dress the wound.

ment and dress it again. This treatment may sound complicated and
tedious, but it is well worth the effort required, because it will free the
patient from the severe problems associated with a wound that refuses
to heal over a long period of time. We have seen several cases of leg
ulcers that had not responded to ointments, powders, or other forms of
treatment over a period of months and even years but that responded to
treatment with horsetail and calendula ointment by closing and healing
(see page 224–228).

ADDITIONAL HERBS FOR THE SPRING CURE

Apart from these three classic blood purifiers, many other wonderful herbs act in a similar fashion or do a fine job of rounding off harsh tastes in your herbal tea mixtures: ramsons (bear's garlic), birch leaves, cowslip flowers, and elder flowers. The last two are sweet, fragrant heralds of spring that can be freshly harvested only for a few short weeks in April or May. Birch leaves are used as a tea only as long as they are tender and light green in color (see page 185). Ramsons is a wild-growing relative of common garlic (with an odor just as intense), and it too can be found only in May. After a month of bloom it disappears completely. A tincture can be made from this herb to reenergize sluggish or weak digestive organs, and its leaves can be picked fresh and diced for use in a delicious salad. The purifying and activating effect of ramsons is truly astounding.

Finally, Swedish Bitters elixir must also be mentioned in this context as a highly effective agent for purifying the blood and cleansing the system. It is best taken in a cup of herbal tea (see chapter 8).

To conclude this chapter on cleansing and purifying, we want to share with you our favorite herbal tea formulas for the annual spring "cure." Of course, you are free to enjoy them at any other time of year as well.

The Fasting Tea is a blend we specifically recommend for use during any type of fasting or slimming cure. Since often blood pressure and circulation are a little shaky during a fasting cure, we have added hawthorn to balance that tendency (see also pages 139–140).

❧ Fasting Tea ❧

4 parts hawthorn flowers with leaves
4 parts stinging nettle leaves
2 parts horsetail
3 parts blackberry leaves
3 parts milk thistle fruit
2 parts goldenrod

Five to six cups per day should be consumed for several weeks, or for a somewhat longer period of time than the fasting or slimming cure itself, since the liver and kidneys will continue to require help even after the cure for the removal of toxins dissolved in the blood.

For people who want to get slimmer we have developed a specific tea that can be combined with almost any program or diet for weight reduction. Its effect is diuretic, flushing, and strongly detoxifying. In contrast to chemical "diet pills," this tea has no harmful side effects whatsoever.

Some people want to lose weight so quickly at any cost that they misuse diuretics, laxatives, and other preparations to a tragic extent. Please bear in mind that the tea formula we recommend is not a wonder cure for becoming thin. In our opinion there is no way around the physiological fact that the body uses up its fat deposits *only when it takes in fewer nutrients than it uses* to sustain its normal functioning, which includes getting rid of waste and excess as well as fueling exercise and activity. If you want to lose weight in the quickest possible manner, take in less and be more active. That is nature's way.

❧ Tea for a Slimming Cure ❧

4 parts birch leaves
4 parts raspberry leaves
3 parts blackthorn flowers
3 parts restharrow root
2 parts artichoke herb
2 parts goldenrod
1 part rose hips
1 part calendula flowers

The daily dosage for this tea mixture should be about five cups.

The use of such a fasting or slimming tea is of particular importance for overweight people who desire to or must reduce their weight for personal or medical reasons, to assist their bodies to diminish and excrete the assembled masses of fat cells together with the toxins and metabolic residues they contain. A metabolism that has literally grown fat and lazy cannot perform this task without subtle, yet effective and continual stimulation. It is well known that the success of a slimming cure is directly dependent on whether the patient accomplishes a general purification, retuning, and revitalization of the body as well as of the mind and emotional state.

The following recipe is for those who feel the need to cleanse their bodies on an ongoing basis. Three to five cups should be drunk each day.

🍃 Blood-Purifying Tea 🍃

5 parts dandelion (including the root)
4 parts raspberry leaves
4 parts stinging nettle leaves
4 parts birch leaves
3 parts elder flowers

This formula makes a wonderful spring tea. It is quite potent, yet it has a delightful aroma especially when prepared from fresh herbs.

For those lucky people who have a clean garden of their very own—and by "clean" we mean free of chemical pesticides and artificial fertilizers and the like—we wholeheartedly recommend cultivating and harvesting springtime herbs yourselves. (See chapter 18.) They are very easy to grow. In most cases it is enough to allow them to flourish just like weeds and pick them fresh to prepare an excellent blood-cleansing tea.

In April, May, and June you'll be able to rise early and walk through your garden before breakfast, picking a few leaves of stinging nettle (best use a garden glove for them), along with leaves from the birch tree and the blackberry bush. You can grab a small handful of hawthorn flowers and a cluster of elder flowers. Each day your mixture can vary. After gathering your morning's harvest, put the herbs into a teapot and pour boiling water over them, then cover and allow them to steep for one to three minutes. Now you can sit back and enjoy one of the most fragrant and delicious cups of tea you've ever tasted. These teas are a blessing for your health: they are stimulating, invigorating, and cleansing as well.

For all three of the above-mentioned tea formulas, it is important to note that they must never be used to eliminate edema (water retention in the body tissues) caused by impaired heart or kidney function.

PROBLEMS WITH BLEMISHED SKIN

Because of the close relationship between the kidneys and the skin and mucous membranes, dealing with the problem of skin blemishes belongs to the area of blood-cleansing cures. Impure skin, difficulties with the complexion, and chronic skin diseases come from within, and though they may be soothed or calmed by the external applications of creams and ointments, they cannot be healed in that manner. The skin disease itself may be considered a symptom of a pathological metabolic problem and very often can be greatly improved by stimulating the detoxi-fying and excretory organs, the liver and the kidneys. Take three to five cups of this tea each day for several weeks.

❧ Tea for Skin Diseases and Blemished Skin ❧

3 parts stinging nettle
3 parts horsetail
3 parts goldenrod
3 parts dandelion root with herb
2 parts white dead nettle flowers
2 parts meadowsweet herb
2 parts yellow bedstraw
1 parts rose hips
1 parts calendula flowers

Although acne is a widespread complexion disorder, it is actually a dif-ferent problem in that it is caused primarily by a hormonal imbalance. This is why, as a general rule, teenage acne disappears after puberty, although it tends to do so as slowly as it came. However, the following tea mixture may be of some help.

❧ Acne Tea ❧

8 parts lady's mantle
6 parts white dead nettle flowers
6 parts wild heartsease (or wild pansy)

If two to three cups of this tea are taken every day for several weeks the complexion should improve considerably.

In most cases of skin disease and abnormality, considerable and timely improvement can be achieved by a change of diet toward fresh, vital foods (such as natural vegetables, fruits, grains, and whole-food products) and away from foods rich in oils and fats, especially saturated fats. A healing fast is perhaps a more radical step, but it usually brings more dramatic results. In either case, a long-term blood-cleansing cure is recommended as well.

❧ 6 ❧

HERBS AND
YOUR IMMUNE SYSTEM

Resist beginnings; the prescription comes too late when the disease has gained strength by long delays.

Remedia Amoris

For a long time the medical world thought that colds—and infectious diseases in general—were caused by the transmission of bacteria and viruses. The result of this scientific assumption was widespread abuse of antibiotics, which caused irreparable harm to the health of people in all the industrialized nations of the world and the United States in particular, even extending to delayed reactions such as *Candida albicans* infections and a tremendous increase in allergies. Even today a wild urge to destroy these "enemy" microorganisms is foremost in the minds of many patients and physicians alike, even though we now know that it is not the presence or absence of microorganisms but rather the state of our defense mechanisms that determines infection. This situation was put in perspective by the nineteenth-century French physiologist Claude Bernard, who said, "The pathogen is nothing, the milieu is everything." This could be paraphrased as follows: It isn't the causative agent that is the decisive factor, but rather the medium in which it is allowed to flourish. In this age of AIDS and cancer, we have at last come to realize that, in both the long and the short run, our health depends on the reactive ability of our immune systems.

57

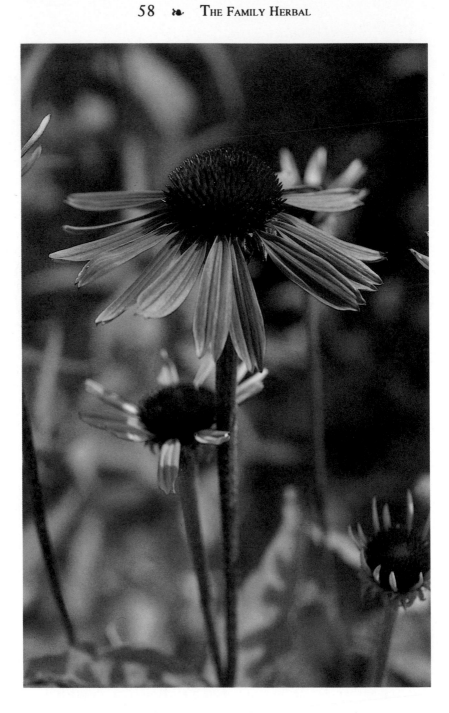

Cone-Flower   *Echinacea purpurea*

Herbologists know a series of medicinal herbs that act specifically to strengthen our body's defense mechanisms. Today, the best-known of these is the cone-flower (*Echinacea purpurea, Echinacea pallida,* and *Echinacea angustifolia*). Other folk names for this lovely garden flower are purple daisy, hedgehog coneflower, and Sampson root. Although this plant is not one of the traditional herbs known to European folk wisdom, we know a great deal about its benefits and acting principles because such intensive research has been done on this remarkable herb over the past few decades. Echinacea is native to the North American continent and was traditionally used by Native American peoples, who applied its roots and leaves to heal all kinds of wounds. To garden lovers echinacea is well known as a decorative garden flower that blooms through most of the year. Today it is also cultivated for medicinal purposes. Either the root alone or the whole plant is extracted fresh, usually in alcohol, because aqueous extracts (tea) do not produce as good results. Echinacea tincture has proved to be a truly natural and effective immuno-stimulant, that is, a substance that fights colds and infections introduced by bacteria, viruses, and fungi indirectly by activating the body's inherent defense reactions. How this works is a fascinating process.

HOW YOUR IMMUNE SYSTEM WORKS

Generally speaking, our immune system is a very precisely working defense system, one that guarantees that the organism is not continuously overflooded with pathogens such as bacteria or viruses. Without it, we could not live, nor would we have any process by which to heal and recover. This is why the most dangerous diseases of our day are those that block, weaken, or destroy the body's own defense system.

Our immune system works via two different defense mechanisms: the specific and the nonspecific. The specific immune system is able to form a specific antibody against a certain invader. It is by virtue of this system's "memory" that in the case of a repeated infection the intruder is immediately recognized and thus can quickly be rendered harmless. This is why we get certain childhood diseases only once. Immunizations also work via this same mechanism: by introducing into the body a weakened form of a specific bacteria or virus, a specific antibody is formed that protects against further "invasions" of that particular infection. So far, so good. Yet the specific immune system has a major disadvantage—

it's slow. In the case of a primary infection, it will not reach its full effectiveness until between five and fourteen days have elapsed!

If the body is invaded by germs that bring the disease to its outbreak within a very short time, as is the case with cold and flu infections, the first symptoms show up within eighteen to forty-eight hours after the onset of infection. It is crucial that the organism be able to wage an intense campaign against these invaders. Only the nonspecific immune system is capable of doing that. Its main agents are special white blood cells, the so-called macrophages. These "killer" cells maintain a constantly vigilant protective force that continuously attacks pathological germs and swallows them up before they amount to any significant threat. The quicker the invaders are eliminated, the less likely is the danger that the disease will come to a head, that is, that pains or complaints will arise. The tricky thing about most viruses that cause head colds and flu is that they constantly change their appearance, that is, their surface structure; hence they do not provoke a specific immune system response, and so require constant defense by the nonspecific immune system.

USE OF ECHINACEA TO ACTIVATE THE NONSPECIFIC IMMUNE SYSTEM

Extensive experimentation with animal subjects and clinical testing has shown that extracts prepared from fresh echinacea herb and root can indeed improve the effectiveness of our immune system defenses. Very often, timely administration of echinacea tincture can boost the body's reactions to a level that completely prevents the onset of symptoms or at least reduces the duration of the infection and/or reduces the impact and intensity of the patient's complaints.

Echinacea For Prevention of Colds and Flu

We should be wise enough to react to any infection as quickly as our front-line white blood cells do by taking echinacea drops to assist them in their battle. Of course, prevention is the best strategy of all—for example, in times of high risk of infection, such as when many people around you are coming down with colds or flu, or when the whole family feels weak or tired due to a sudden change to cold or rainy weather.

Numerous scientific studies done in Germany during the last few years have shown that combined preparations with echinacea are superior to medications consisting of echinacea tincture or extract alone. We have achieved our best results with a homeopathic mixture we call Flu and Cold tincture. It combines echinacea mother-tincture with five other homeopathic herbal dilutions. (Since the preparation of this formula must be reserved for the pharmacist or professional homeopath, we give here, as an exception, the exact gram measurement. You should be able to obtain the ready-made formula in your health food store.)

❧ Flu and Cold Tincture ❧

Echinacea angustifolia (10 g per 100 g tincture)
3x Aconitum
3x Belladonna
3x Eupatorium perfoliatum
3x Adonis vernalis
1x Myristica sebifera

As the success of this natural medication depends more than in others upon the right application and the right timing, we advise you to strictly abide by the following directions: As soon as you become aware of any initial symptoms like a sudden chill, a headache, a sore throat, or repeated sneezing, immediately take 50 drops. It is of utter importance not to wait another hour but to act immediately. Then, continue with 20 drops every hour. Depending upon how you feel, continue this dosage for about two days (except at nights—you'd better sleep), and then gradually reduce to three times per day until all symptoms have disappeared. Then stop taking the medication! This too is important, for it has been found that a so-called interval therapy is more successful than continuous use of the echinacea preparation. The next time you again feel endangered by an infection or flu, you should take the drops again. Once an infection has grown to full bloom and the patient must lie in bed with a high fever, it seems that the echinacea medication cannot help anymore.

The simplest way to take the drops is to place them in a glass or cup with a very small amount of water. Some people drop them directly into the mouth under the tongue. In either case, it is best to keep the tincture in your mouth for ten to twenty seconds before swallowing. This allows it to be absorbed by the mucous membranes within the mouth cavity and thus to enter your system more quickly and thoroughly. If you are using the tincture as a prevention before infection has set on, take

20 drops three times each day. Also, when you are traveling and you are exposed to dramatic changes in climate and temperature, you'll always be on the safe side if you have your echinacea tincture at hand.

Thanks to the intense scientific discussion about this herb, it is now established as a fact that preparations with echinacea—whether homeopathic or allopathic—are excellent immune boosters for the prophylaxis and therapy of recurrent infections of the upper respiratory tract and the urinary passageways (the latter subject is discussed on pages 197–198) as well as for chronic inflammatory processes.

Our Own Experience

In the past few years we have had tremendous success in giving echinacea preparations to our children whenever they reported that many of their classmates were having the flu or were missing from school or kindergarten. We haven't had a real case of the flu in our family during all these years.

Many years ago I (Peter) used to be very susceptible to flu when I was under a lot of stress. Almost every time I needed to prepare for an important business trip and had to work around the clock to get ready, I would experience various cold symptoms such as head congestion, fever blisters on the lips, feverish chills, or that general "down" feeling. Over time I learned how to deal with the situation. In the beginning, it took me a whole week to ward off the unwanted symptoms. Later I needed only three or four days, then only one day to overcome this weakness. Today, with the help of echinacea tincture, which I keep always at the ready, I can handle intense periods of stress very well without being forced by my immune system to slow down or curtail my activities.

Psychoimmunology

American scientists have recently established the fact that intense physical or emotional stress negatively influences our immune system. On the other hand, recent studies have also clearly demonstrated that a depressed and inactive immune system, such as that found in cancer patients, can be vitalized and energized by certain thought patterns and positive feelings. It is no longer just a science fiction fantasy to intensely imagine your own white blood cells surrounding "an enemy virus," or sending out "white light" (white blood cells?) to dissolve and destroy cancer cells.

This is in truth advanced psychoimmunology, which in turn can be effectively supported and enhanced by herbal medicinals!

ADDITIONAL REMEDIES FOR COLDS AND FLU

Colds and flu are heralded by such symptoms as runny nose, aching throat, hoarseness, coughing, back pain, aching muscles, and a general feeling of fatigue. In children particularly, these conditions may be accompanied by earache or high fever. Besides echinacea, there are of course other herbs and procedures that can strengthen the body's immune system. We recommend a special Cold Tea along with an herbal footbath or a thyme full bath.

🐚 Cold Tea For Adults 🐚

6 parts ephedra herb
3 parts elder flowers
3 parts rose hips
2 parts willow bark
2 parts linden flowers
2 parts chamomile flowers
2 parts hawthorn leaves with flowers

🐚 Cold Tea For Children 🐚

4 parts linden flowers
4 parts mullein
4 parts elder flowers
4 parts rose hips
4 parts thyme

This second tea has an anti-inflammatory effect and promotes sweating, which is one of the classical means by which you can prevent a cold from taking hold. Children love the taste of this tea, especially when it is sweetened with a little honey.

Flu Footbath

When you've gotten your feet thoroughly soaked in the cold and feel frozen through and through, nothing takes away the shivering like a hot footbath with linden and elder flowers. Simply mix ½ cup of each of the two herbs together and prepare a hot water infusion. After steeping it for ten minutes, pour the extract into a wash tub or large bucket and fill it with hot water (as hot as you enjoy) up to the level of your calves. Immerse your feet for about ten to fifteen minutes; you will experience both delight and relief. Then lightly dry your feet and slip into a pair of soft, thick woolen socks.

Today, we recognize that there are highly sensitive points located on the soles of our feet, so-called reflex points or zones, which can be activated and vitalized by massage or thermal stimulation. These reflex zones correspond to all the various vital organs of our body. Therefore it hardly comes as a surprise that defense-strengthening herbs act very strongly on the entire organism via the soles of our feet, an effect that often surpasses that of drinking a tea. Ideally you can combine the two therapies by drinking an elder-linden flower tea while having the foot bath. Both herbs and applications will cause considerable sweating, and this is the important thing, for sweating is a natural mechanism for discharging toxins. You must allow your body to rest after completing the footbath; give it time to respond to the treatment.

Linden Flowers

The linden or lime tree (*Tilia platyphyllos* and *Tilia cordata*) is very common throughout Europe and through the ages has been the subject of many poems and romantic songs and much folklore. This beautiful tree has been revered since pagan times. Today, it is a familiar symbol in European literature and art, representing both masculine strength and power and the feminine qualities of contemplation and receptiveness.

The healing power hidden in the lovely blossoms of both species may be tapped by harvesting the flowers when the majority of the blossoms on the tree have just opened, usually in June. At that point they contain their highest concentration of active ingredients. Among the distinctive aspects of these flowers are their marvelously sweet scent and the parchmentlike bract growing at the top of each flower cluster.

Elder Flowers

The elder (*Sambucus nigra*) is another traditional garden plant that has found its way into many legends and fairy tales. In ancient times, the elder was held to be the dwelling of the house spirits, and to this day it can be found on almost every farm in northern Europe, often right next to the stable or barn. The elder can grow quite tall and often looks more like

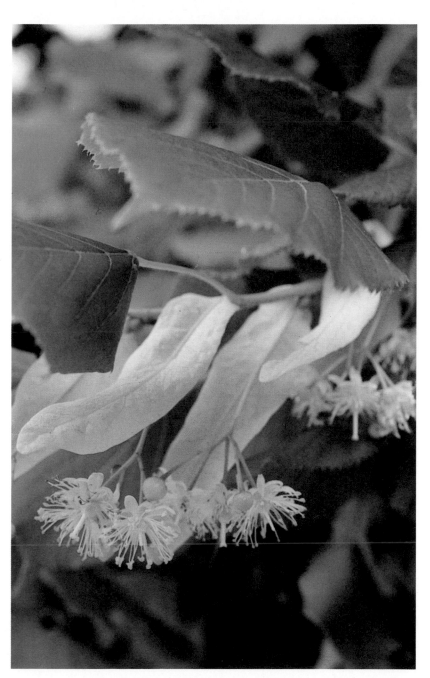

LINDEN FLOWERS *Tilla platyphyllos*

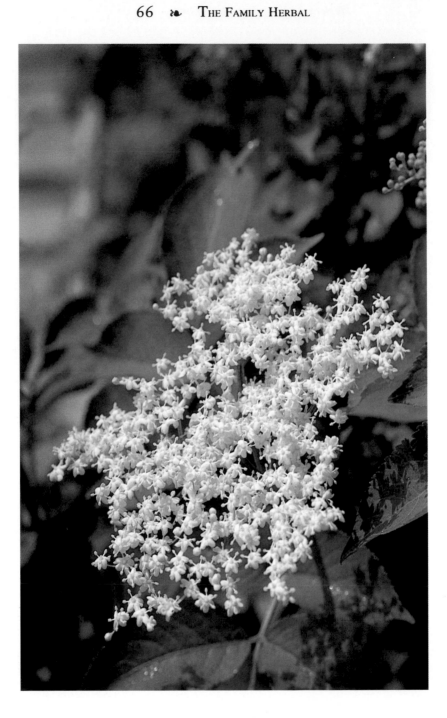

ELDER FLOWERS *Sambucus nigra*

a small tree than a shrub. Its large, flat flower umbel, dotted with tiny whitish blossoms in May and June, exudes a peculiar, intensely bitter-sweet scent. If you don't harvest the flowers in the spring for either a "sweating" or a cold tea, or to make elder syrup or elder pop (see pages 249–250), small black berries—a favorite food for many birds—will form in the fall. These berries can be eaten raw and are praised by herbalists for their high concentration of vitamins and minerals. They do have a slight laxative effect, so it's best to enjoy them in moderate amounts. (When preserved by canning, however, the berries do not have this effect.) Elderberries make a delicious and healthful dessert, especially when combined with plums or pears (which ripen at the same time of year).

Medicinal Effects of Linden and Elder Flowers

Linden and elder flowers are almost always used together, because their effects are so very similar. Both are excellent herbs for colds and flu. When taken as a tea, they stimulate the body's defense mechanisms and cause the organs to detoxify by initiating the process of sweating. R. F. Weiss, in his classic herbal textbook *Lehrbuch der Phytotherapie,* describes a clinical study, conducted by two pediatricians in Chicago, of children with severe cold symptoms. Fifty-five children were treated with bed rest, linden flower tea, and one to two aspirin tablets. A second group of thirty-seven children received the same therapy but with the addition of sulfonamides. A third group, comprising sixty-seven children, received antibiotics only. To the great surprise of the physicians and their supporting staff, the children treated with bed rest and linden flower tea recovered most quickly with the lowest incidence of complications (such as infections of the middle ear). The two groups that received chemical therapy required longer recovery time and also suffered more complications.

The tea from fresh or dried linden and elder blossoms should be drunk as hot as possible. The process of sweating will begin only after two or three cups of the tea have been consumed. (Incidentally, two cups taken fifteen to thirty minutes before you enter a sauna will help you sweat more easily.) This lovely-tasting, fine-smelling tea is a favorite with children and babies, especially when sweetened with a teaspoon of honey. In times of heightened risk of infection, it can be given morning and evening.

Thyme Bath

Another old and highly reliable treatment for nipping colds and flu in the bud is the thyme bath. Thyme (*Thymus vulgaris*), besides being a familiar culinary herb, is one of the oldest medicinal plants we know. Indigenous to the Mediterranean, where it grows on dry, rocky soil and thrives in the blazing sun, thyme was highly prized as a healing agent in ancient times, especially by the Greek physicians Hippocrates, Theophrastus, and Dioscurides. In the Middle Ages, the plant was lauded by the alchemist Albertus Magnus and by Hildegard of Bingen. For centuries it has been carefully cultivated in monastery gardens. Its mucus-dissolving and expectorant effect in the treatment of cough and bronchitis has been proved by modern science. Its antispasmodic effect is also generally recognized in the treatment of whooping cough. Used as a bath, it has an additional nerve-strengthening effect and is quite beneficial for inflammatory skin problems as well.

For a full thyme bath, brew an extremely strong infusion using two cups of dried thyme and two quarts of boiling water. Allow the covered mixture to steep for ten minutes; drain off the extract and pour it into the bathtub, then fill the tub with more hot water at body temperature (about 98° F, or 37° C). (See illustration, page 37.) Do not expect to fall asleep immediately after taking the bath; lie down wrapped in your bathrobe or a number of warm towels and bury yourself under the covers. Let your body rest while you continue perspiring—about thirty to sixty minutes will do. This is extremely important; without this second phase of the therapy, the entire process would be to no avail. You should not take this bath more than once a day.

During the bath the essential oils are released by the hot water, because they are quite volatile. Not only are they absorbed by the pores of the skin, but at the same time the ambient steam reaches the inflamed mucous membranes via the upper respiratory tract and there unfolds its antibacterial effect. Children suffering from bronchitis, asthma, or a barking cough react extremely well to thyme baths. Such an herbal bath can be surprisingly effective, as the body absorbs the active substances through the skin over the entire surface of the body, instead of through the intestinal tract as with oral treatments.

TREATING FEVER NATURALLY

When a full-blown cold is accompanied by fever, we should take this as

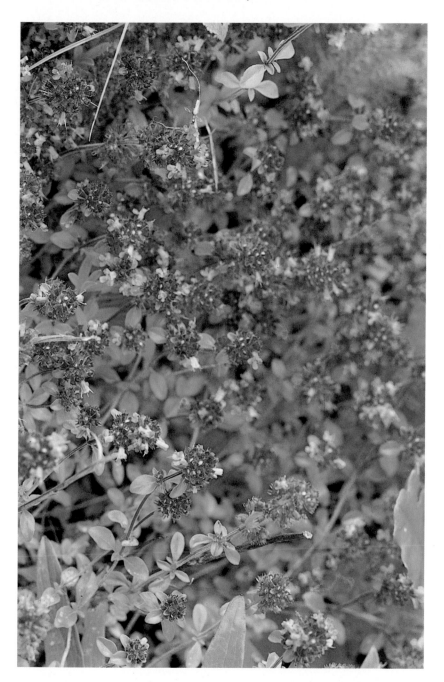

THYME   *Thymus vulgaris*

a positive sign that the immune system is functioning properly. Fever is one of our bodies' most effective defense reactions. By the increase in body temperature of one to five degrees Fahrenheit (two to three degrees Centigrade), viruses and germs are destroyed and the healing process becomes initiated. That is why suppressing a fever is the last thing you should do! In natural cancer therapy, physicians artificially induce fever in order to activate the immune system. Yet it often happens that physicians receive midnight calls from worried parents requesting some medicinal agent to immediately lower their child's fever. Perhaps these parents are doing themselves a favor by preventing the child from waking up every hour during the night, but such therapy doesn't do the child any good at all. Its direct consequence is that the defense system of the child, which is operating at full steam, becomes undermined. This is detrimental in the long run, as babies and children are still in the initial process of "stocking" their immune systems. So please be assured that a fever of 103° or even 104° F (40° C), which is often considered to be quite high in the United States, is entirely purposeful and need not be lowered. (You will naturally notice if other signs of serious illness during an episode of fever indicate the need to contact a doctor.)

Compresses to Lower Fever

If the child's temperature rises over 104° F (40° C) and remains there for more than twelve hours, a physician must be consulted. If the fever unduly burdens the entire organism, it can be diverted by the age-old method of applying wet compresses around the lower legs, without the self-healing capacity of the body being adversely affected. To do this, dip two linen or cotton cloths (dish towels work well) in cold water, wring them out, and wrap them around the patient's calves, covering as wide an area as possible between the ankle and the knee (see figure 5). A dry linen cloth is applied on top, followed by a wrapping of terry cloth or woolen cloth. Securing the cloths is not necessary so long as the patient keeps his or her legs still. Leave the compress on for about twenty minutes (by which time it will be warm and beginning to dry out) and repeat the procedure. Compresses are always applied simultaneously to both lower legs. (Not at all incidentally, we find this traditional method of treatment far more effective than the practice of sponging down the entire body.) The treatment can be discontinued as soon as the patient's temperature has dropped to 101° F (38.5° C). Note one cardinal rule, however: the feet

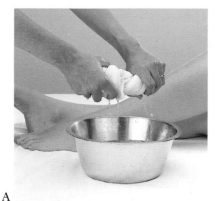

A

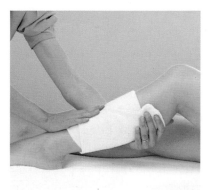

B

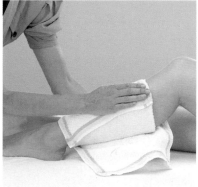

C

FIGURE 5

**Calf Compress to
Lower Fever**

A. Dip two small linen towels (dish towels) in cool water and wring out.
B. Wrap a towel around each calf.
C. Cover each compress with a dry linen or cotton towel (dish towel), followed by a small terry cloth towel.

must be warm before applying the compresses. *Never administer treatments involving cold water to parts of the body that are already cold!*

For a simplified form of the lower-leg compress, dip cotton or wool socks in cold water, squeeze the water out, and put them on. Put on a dry pair of larger-sized socks over the wet compress socks. Repeat the procedure as soon as the coolness in the stockings has dissipated.

Food and Drink for Feverish Conditions

People used to believe that eating during an acute infection was the way to regain strength. Today, we know that a lack of appetite can be a very wise reaction. This is the body's way of automatically switching to a fasting mode so that it can concentrate all its efforts on fighting the infection. We would do well to recognize this lack of appetite as the body's way to conserve energy by not allowing the extra work of digestion to burden or deplete its resources. When your organism is "over the worst," it automatically regains its appetite with a craving for raw fruits and vegetables. These foods contain the vitamins and minerals that the body urgently needs; they also stimulate digestion and provide the body with the roughage needed to cleanse the system. As soon as you notice real improvement in the patient's general feeling, detoxifying teas should be administered (such as those listed in chapter 5). Chewing a small amount of comb honey can also provide the body with a large quantity of vital nutritious substances.

Although feverish patients may not have any appetite at all, they make up for this by being quite thirsty. They can safely be given rose hip tea (with a little honey) and stinging nettle tea (also with a little honey and a spot of lemon juice), or else fruit juices rich in vitamin C. The absolutely best drink for strengthening a patient's immune system is one or two glasses of freshly squeezed red beet juice along with the same amount of fresh carrot juice. (Note: a few drops of vegetable oil or cream must be added to chemically bind the carotenoids in the carrot juice so that they can be better absorbed by the intestines.)

BATHS FOR INCREASING BODY TEMPERATURE

If a cold is *not* accompanied by fever, it is advisable to support the body's fight against it by temporarily raising the body temperature. Three methods have proved to be most successful: the sauna or steam bath, the so-called Schlenz bath, and the increasing temperature foot bath. Sauna and steam baths, with various herbal additives, have been successfully used for thousands of years by such peoples as the Eskimos, Finns, Native Americans, and Japanese. They are just as effective today as they were in ancient times for toughening the organism and for supporting the treatment of colds. If the sauna or steam bath is augmented by essential oils of thyme, sage, pine needles, or dwarf pine, these oils will act directly on the mucous membranes of the upper respiratory tract. By the way, you will have a more effective sauna if you drink one or two cups of linden flower tea beforehand.

The Schlenz bath (named for its founder, Maria Schlenz), or increasing temperature bath, is actually an intensification of the full bath described on pages 67–68. First, the bath temperature is 98° F (36.5° C); it is gradually increased over time to 102° F (39° C) by slowly adding hot water. The bath should last between thirty and sixty minutes (twenty to thirty minutes for children). The temperature of the bath must not be allowed to drop. While sitting in the tub, you can massage your skin with a brush or loofah sponge until it turns red. This massage acts along with the duration of the bath to leach the skin and thus strongly activates the excretory processes of the skin. As in the case of the thyme bath, go to bed directly afterward. Rest and sweat! Adding thyme or dwarf pine oil to the water amplifies the effect.

Since the Schlenz bath is quite strenuous for the circulatory system, especially for older persons, some people may prefer the so-called temperature-increasing footbath. It is based on the same principle, yet does not put as much stress on the heart and circulatory system. The temperature of the footbath is gradually increased as well and must not be allowed to drop off. The bathing time lasts from ten to fifteen minutes. Afterward the feet need to be kept warm, and the entire body needs time to sweat.

Warning: All three of these natural stimulation therapies—steam bath or sauna, Schlenz bath, and temperature-increasing footbath—are advisable only for generally healthy individuals. Patients with cardiovascular problems should not undertake them without consulting their physician first.

❧ 7 ❧

TREATING THE "COMMON" COLD—NATURALLY

Medicus curat, natura sanat—The physician treats, but nature heals.

Hippocrates

Acute head cold sometimes occurs as the first symptom of a general cold, which may include coughing, congestion, aching, fever, swollen glands, and sore throat. In some instances the head cold may be the only sign of an infection. It involves inflammation of the mucous membranes in the nose, sinuses, and nasal cavities, which become swollen and discharge a large quantity of secretion. That's why your nose feels stopped up, your breathing difficult, and your head congested. If this is the case, it is advisable to use a mild nose ointment that will—at least for a short time—soothe the irritated mucous membranes and open up your nasal passages.

A cold is really a very minor thing, but it may develop into a monumental problem if not cured properly and in a timely manner. During our numerous flights to and from other countries, we have experienced that an uncured sinus infection can cause excruciating headaches during the landing, because pressure cannot be equalized in the cavities of the head. Chronic irritation of the nasal cavities and sinuses, or even a suppurative condition of these cavities, can turn into a constant source of disturbance to the lymphatic and immune systems, as well as a perpetual source of headaches. This is why it is very well worth going to the trouble of carefully and completely healing a nasal infection.

CHEMICAL NASAL SPRAYS
VERSUS NATUROPATHIC METHODS

By all means, stay away from chemical-based nasal sprays, as these often have devastating side effects. Such sprays contain a complex of active ingredients (alpha-sympathomimetic agents) that cause local constriction of the blood vessels, thus preventing excess secretion. The catch is that this effect cannot be limited to the blood vessels in the mucous membranes of the nose. The chemical agents eventually end up in the respiratory and gastrointestinal tract, and result in a systematic constriction of the blood vessels throughout the entire body, consequently increasing both blood pressure and pulse rate—which is about the worst condition to impose on a body suffering from a heavy cold or fever. Other side effects are irritation and frequently an overcompensating drying-out of the mucous membranes in the nose itself. We have seen cases in which the sense of smell and taste were considerably impaired for a long time after application. Only after repeated flushings with mallow tea could status quo functioning be reestablished in these cases. Because they are capable of causing dramatic spasms in the respiratory tract, nasal sprays of this type can be dangerous for babies and small children.

The widespread advocacy of nasal sprays provides a perfect example of the short-sighted, mechanistic approach favored by the medical establishment. In the view of this system, if the secretion given off by the mucous membranes is overactivated, a chemical agent must be administered to stop it immediately. The point that is conveniently forgotten or, at the least, played down is that it is impossible to limit the effects of such an agent to a specific area of the body. (This is also true of antibiotics.) In naturopathy, on the other hand, the self-regulatory mechanism of the body is never undermined in favor of a fast symptomatic result. In this example, the excess production of mucus and its secretion serves to cleanse the respiratory tract, ridding it of unwanted bacteria and viruses. Naturopathy tackles the problem in a relatively roundabout manner (nonspecific stimulation therapies), in order to induce and support the body to counteract the "invader" in its own way. Taking shortcuts by administering heavy-duty chemical agents makes it possible to achieve local and immediate results, yet in the long run this approach weakens the body's natural defense mechanisms, causing them ultimately to break down completely after decades and generations of being bombarded by chemical warfare.

REMEDIES FOR CONGESTION

In our opinion, a good natural nose ointment should contain the essential oils of eucalyptus, peppermint, pine needles, dwarf pine, and possibly camphor. This can be a great help, especially for children who are having trouble falling asleep because they cannot breathe properly. For babies, for whom the severe head cold is most dramatic because it interferes with both sleeping and nursing, we recommend putting a few drops of eucalyptus oil on the child's pillow, bed sheets, and covers. (Laundering will remove any traces of the oil.) Setting up a room humidifier near the baby's bed and adding ten to twenty drops of this oil to the water is also very beneficial. A mild chest rub containing the above-mentioned essential oils as well as cypress oil, sage oil, and lavender oil can be rubbed on your baby's chest after he or she is six months old. Such an ointment alleviates the congestion of secretions in the nose during sleep, as well as inhibiting bacteria deep down in the bronchial tubes while warming the entire chest from the inside out. Ointments and chest rubs that contain menthol should not be used for babies, because menthol can irritate the skin, eyes, and mucosa.

We consider it extremely important, especially when treating babies and small children, not only that natural and correctly dosed active ingredients be used, but also that the secondary or base ingredients of an ointment be made of pure, natural substances. (Vegetable oils and beeswax are ideal for this purpose; check product labels when shopping for these ointments in health food stores or pharmacies.)

Inhalation Therapy

In the treatment of both head and chest congestion, a chest rub ointment of the type described above is also very practical for inhalation therapy. Simply dissolve a teaspoon of the balm in a bowl containing hot water, sit down at the bowl with a bath towel pulled up over your head, and breathe in the vapors. Please keep the eyes closed during this

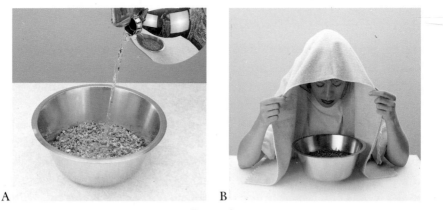

A   B

FIGURE 6

Chamomile Steam Inhalation

A. Place chamomile flowers into a bowl   B. Drape a bath towel over the head and
    and pour boiling water over them.   inhale the hot vapors with eyes closed.

process to protect them from irritation (see figure 6). Inhalation treatment should be carried out for no longer than ten to fifteen minutes, and no oftener than twice a day. You will find that the beneficial and soothing effect of this treatment is astounding!

Chamomile Vapor Inhalation

Another proven method for treating sinus infection is the inhalation of chamomile infusion. Place a handful of chamomile flowers in a bowl and pour boiling water over them. Put a bath towel over your head so that it forms a little tent, and breathe in the hot vapors (see figure 6). Make sure you don't burn yourself in the beginning by letting your face get too close to the bowl. It's better to wait one or two minutes and test the temperature gradually. By the way, this same procedure can also be used to cleanse the complexion, especially in the case of those suffering from skin eruptions, acne, and related skin problems. The chamomile-laden steam opens up the pores and has an antibacterial effect that heals minor skin infections and pimples. German chamomile in particular has a remarkably soothing, anti-inflammatory, and antispasmodic effect, especially in connection with infections of the skin and mucous membrane. (For more on chamomile, see pages 195–199.)

TREATMENT OF BRONCHITIS

Another persistent problem in connection with colds and flu is bronchitis and cough. Herbologists are familiar with a whole series of time-tested and scientifically documented herbs for these problems: plantain, mallow, mullein, coltsfoot, marshmallow, thyme, licorice, cowslip, Iceland moss, and elm bark. When you have just come down with bronchitis, you should use anti-inflammatory herbs that specifically inhibit bacterial growth as well as coat and protect inflamed mucous membranes. Such preparations will alleviate the continuous and torturous urge to cough. A good cough tea mixture with this objective is the following:

❧ Cough Tea No. 1 ☙

8 parts plantain leaves
8 parts coltsfoot flowers
2 parts marshmallow root
2 parts mallow

Coltsfoot

Coltsfoot (*Tussilago farfara*) is one of the earliest spring herbs. Its bright yellow blossoms often peek through patches of sunlit snow as early as February and March. The flowers emerge from stubby, scaly stems and are often buried beneath the still-brown grass or between rocks and stones. Large, heart-shaped leaves with serrated edges and whitish undersides develop long after the flowers. Coltsfoot prefers loamy soil and often thrives on railroad embankments, at the edges of landfills, and on slopes bordering on fields and dirt roads. The flowers (in February and March) and the leaves (in May and June) are harvested almost exclusively from the wild.

The botanical name *Tussilago* derives from the Latin word *tussis* ("cough"), for this herb has been used since the earliest of times to treat that condition. The plant's healing properties come from the combination of bitter ingredients and mucins. The mucins alleviate the severe urge to cough by coating and thus protecting inflamed bronchial mucosa. Coltsfoot helps dissolve and discharge phlegm in cases of chronic bronchitis or silicosis. Also, coltsfoot is recommended in all cases of catarrh (inflammation) of the mouth and throat cavity.

Coltsfoot leaves and flowers are almost always mixed with other

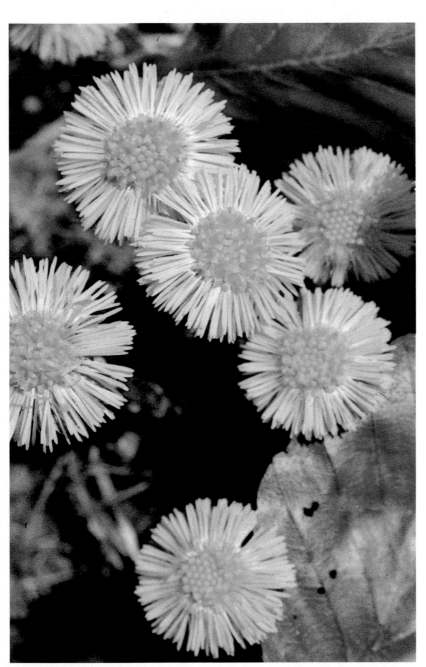

COLTSFOOT   *Tussilago farfara*

"cough herbs" in tea blends—and rightly so, for coltsfoot can have some unwanted side effects when overdosed. The safety of coltsfoot altogether was even questioned in Germany in 1988 because the herb contains pyrrolizidine alkaloids (a toxic chemical compound recently found in a few medicinal plants). Yet, although medical doctors and pharmacists have been irritated and the German Health Authority has imposed restrictions, the risk-benefit evaluation of this medicinal herb still favors its application for acute initial conditions of bronchitis as long as it is not applied for longer than four to six weeks (which will almost never be necessary anyway). A mixture like the one on the previous page can be used without any danger provided it is not applied all year long.

In the advanced stages of bronchitis it is important to loosen and dissolve phlegm so that it can be discharged from the body through coughing. Bear in mind that the almost uncontrollable urge to cough is a useful reaction, for by these abrupt spasms of the bronchioles and the bronchial tubes the body conveys the phlegm that has blocked the respiratory system upward and outward. The important thing is not to suppress the urge to cough (as by taking cough medicines that contain powerful drugs such as codeine) but rather to aid the body in carrying the natural healing process to its rightful conclusion. The following tea is designed to achieve this end.

❧ Cough Tea No. 2 ❧

6 parts thyme
4 parts anise seed
4 parts cowslip root
4 parts mullein
2 parts licorice root

Mullein

Mullein (*Verbascum densiflorum* and *Verbascum phlomoides*) is one of the best-known mucin-containing "cough herbs." In German, mullein is called *Wollblume* ("wool flower") because of the velvety or woolly surface of its hairy leaves. Most of these form a densely packed rosette near the soil, while only a few leaves appear along the single upright stem. The English common name "torchweed" describes this stately plant well. In former times people actually used mullein to make torches by dipping the long, tough stem in wax or pitch.

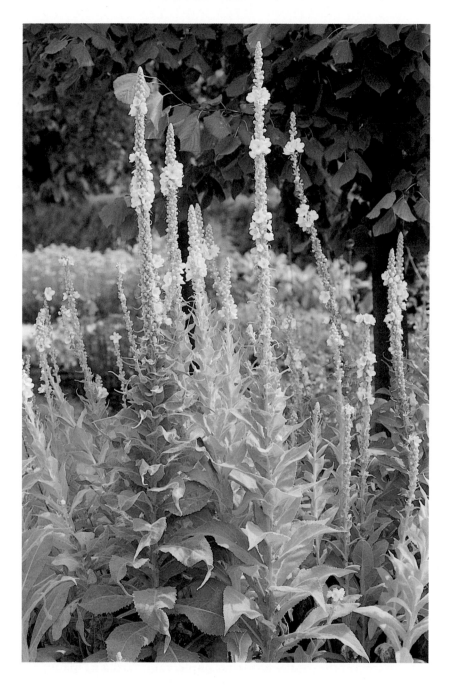

MULLEIN *Verbascum densiflorum*

The plant's yellow, five-petaled flowers sit tightly around the single stem. Occasionally a second stem will emerge from the first, but only at a considerable height. The flowers do not blossom all at the same time, but develop continuously, proceeding up the stem. If mullein finds a comfortable, sunny spot on a grassy slope, it can grow to a height of six feet or more.

If this biennial medicinal herb establishes itself on your property, you will do well to spare it from the lawnmower so that you can harvest the flowers from the stem in August of the plant's second year of growth. The mucins contained in mullein help to heal coughs and alleviate inflammations of the mucuous membrane of the upper respiratory tract. The herb also contains saponines, which aid in dissolving phlegm and encourage expectoration. Mullein flowers are ideally combined in tea mixtures with other herbs that offer similar healing benefits.

We have achieved wonderful results with another cough tea, one that combines both these features (alleviation of the urge to cough and dissolution of phlegm) and also treats hoarseness at the same time:

❧ Cough Tea No. 3 ☙

4 parts plantain
4 parts coltsfoot leaves
3 parts elm bark
3 parts knotgrass
2 parts mallow flowers
1 parts thyme
1 parts licorice root
1 part star anise
1 parts eucalyptus leaves

Plantain

Plantain (*Plantago lanceolata*), one of the major cough medicinals, has a very interesting history. Since the most ancient times it has been one of the medicinal treasures of the peoples of southern Europe and the Germanic tribes. In a classic herbal text of the eleventh century, the healer Macer described the medicinal effects of plantain, listing its many therapeutic uses, including the application of crushed leaves to fresh wounds to actually stop bleeding. That this is no exaggeration has been shown by recent scientific research, because along with other substances plan-

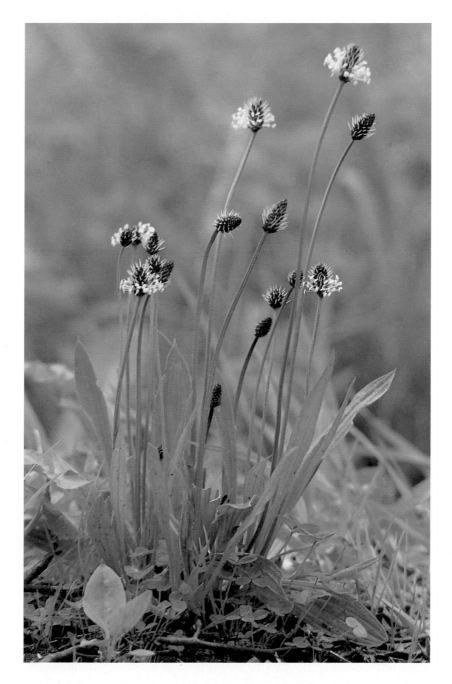

PLANTAIN   *Plantago lanceolata*

tain contains silicic acid, carotinoids, and aucubin, all substances known to promote the coagulation of blood and the quick healing of wounds.

When Europeans "conquered" the New World, the native people of North America referred to the various species of plantain as "the trail left by the white man," because the plants seemed to follow the settlers everywhere. Its seed, which becomes quite sticky when wet, attached itself to shoes, boots, animal hooves, and wagon wheels and was thus spread across the land. Plantain is capable of becoming firmly rooted in the hardest ground, and as a result it can prevail even in highly frequented and trafficked places. In addition, its leaves are extremely tough and cannot be easily crushed or destroyed underfoot. We have even seen plantain growing out of tar streets and concrete surfaces, fighting its way to the light in environments where no other plant would survive.

Plantain by itself represents a comprehensive cough remedy because it protects the mucous membranes, reduces the urge to cough, dissolves mucus, and inhibits bacterial growth and inflammation. Its healing power is optimally utilized when a tea made with plantain as the main ingredient (see Cough Teas 1 and 3, above) is combined with plantain cough syrup and possibly with fresh-squeezed juice from the plantain leaves.

Chest Rub Compresses

In treating bronchitis and throat infection, it is advisable to rub the patient's chest, back, and neck with a natural chest balm that is left on overnight (see figure 7). In using chest rubs, it is imperative that the entire upper body be kept warm afterward by wrapping the patient's chest and upper body with warm towels or a woolen scarf, or by putting on a light woolen undershirt. This thorough warming of the chest in conjunction with simultaneous inhalation of essential oils via the upper respiratory passages is very effective and usually brings relief that lasts through the night.

Cough Syrups for Children

Plantain is often also made into a natural cough syrup that contains plantain extract in relatively high concentration. Of course, you should not use any cough syrup flavored with refined white sugar. A far superior natural sweetener would be honey, beet syrup, or maple syrup. Cough syrup is especially popular with children because it tastes so good. When one of our children has a cough, we never manage to give cough

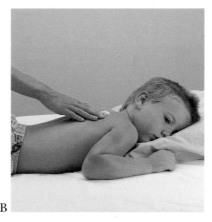

A

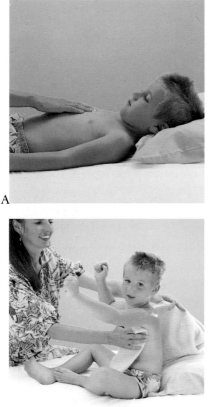

B

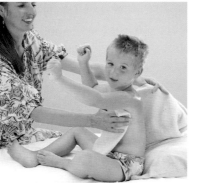

C

FIGURE 7
Chest Compress
A. Rub the chest with a thick layer of natural chest balm.
B. Rub the upper back.
C. Wrap the upper body with a warm terry cloth towel or woolen scarf and fasten to secure in place.

syrup to just that child—each of the others demands a spoonful too!

Combining the Treatments

In the case of a fully developed bronchitis and persistent cough, it is wise to combine the various methods described above and in the previous chapter. To achieve fast, effective relief without interfering with the body's natural defense reactions, administer echinacea drops continuously, cough tea throughout the day, cough syrup every other hour, a thyme bath in the evening, and a chest rub compress overnight.

CHRONIC BRONCHITIS

Bronchitis is one of those conditions that can develop into a chronic problem if it is not completely healed. Children who have been susceptible to coughs for years can be dramatically helped by spending an extended time in the mountains or at the seaside. Chronic bronchitis, or so-called old age cough, often becomes entrenched in older people and, of course, particularly in smokers. Such individuals cannot start the day without going through a prolonged coughing spell until the viscous phlegm has been loosened and the lungs become at least partially cleared. In cases of chronic bronchitis, teas made of cowslip roots and flowers or a mixture of anise seeds and Iceland moss have proven especially effective.

When used in this tea formula, the anise seeds must be crushed before making the infusion (as described on pages 211–212). The cowslip tea is best prepared as a cold infusion from one teaspoon of roots and one cup of water. After standing overnight (approximately eight hours), the mixture is boiled for a moment and steeped for five minutes. Then the tea is ready to drink. The only people who should not use this tea are those with primrose (Primula) allergy. For both teas, two to three cups per day is the proper dosage. (For the use of cowslip flowers, see page 204.)

TREATING SORE THROAT

Colds and flu are often accompanied by "strep throat," or septic sore throat, characterized by an aching sore throat (especially when swallowing), reddening, swelling, and in some cases suppuration of the tonsils and the soft palate. Secondary symptoms are always sensitivity to pressure, enlargement and hardening of the lymph nodes at the corner of the jaw, and often fever. Pain is often deflected to the ears, and infection of the middle ear is frequently present. The ears, nasal passages, and throat cavity are very closely connected, for together with the lymph nodes in the head and neck they form the so-called first line of defense against infection. They can literally be imagined as the outer wall of a fort. If the invaders (bacteria, viruses, etc.) are stopped at this wall and conquered, there is no possibility of them proceeding past this line to endanger the vital organs of the body.

Throat Compresses

A throat compress is recommended when a throat infection is accompanied by sweating or fever. Soak a linen cloth in cold water, wring it out, and apply it around the neck, smoothing it out as much as possible. Wrap a woolen scarf around your neck on top of the compress. After twenty to thirty minutes the compress will be partially dried out and warm and should be removed (as in the procedure for the calf compress, see page 52). A throat compress using Swedish Bitters is even more effective. The directions on pages 105–107 must be followed carefully. These compresses are very effective forms of stimulation therapy and may be applied several times a day safely and comfortably. However, a very serious case of strep throat should be monitored by a physician.

Sage

The choice remedy for countering throat infection is sage (*Salvia officinalis*), an anti-inflammatory herb that inhibits bacterial growth and acts as a disinfectant, particularly by virtue of its essential oil. It is the herb for all infections of the mucous membrane of the mouth, throat, and gums. Bleeding and shrinking of the gums, as well as pressure sores caused by dentures, can be improved significantly by rinsing the mouth with sage tea. Sage is also a very effective mouthwash to eliminate bad breath.

In addition, sage is employed in the treatment of gastroenteritis (inflammation of the small intestine and the stomach) as an antispasmodic remedy for relieving flatulence and assuaging pain. A cup of sage tea several times a day, preferably taken half an hour before meals, can bring about instant relief. *However, this tea should be drunk only as needed and not over an extended period of time!* Sage is also a favorite culinary herb in fine cuisine. Spaghetti made with fresh sage leaves is a favorite in our house, and this delicious ingredient can easily be grown in your own garden.

Many species of sage exist; however, only *Salvia officinalis* and *Salvia Montana* are useful for medicinal purposes. Sage was probably brought by the Romans from the Mediterranean across the Alps to central Europe. In the Middle Ages, it was carefully cultivated in monastery herb gardens and was highly esteemed. In 1688, a 414-page book exclusively about this herb appeared.

To treat sore throat with sage, make a tea from either fresh or dried sage leaves and let it steep for five minutes. When it has cooled somewhat, take a cup of the tea and gargle with it extensively. The beneficial feeling of constriction of the throat, often perceived by children as unpleasant, can be lessened by making the tea from half sage leaves and half chamomile flowers. This gargling has to be repeated every one to

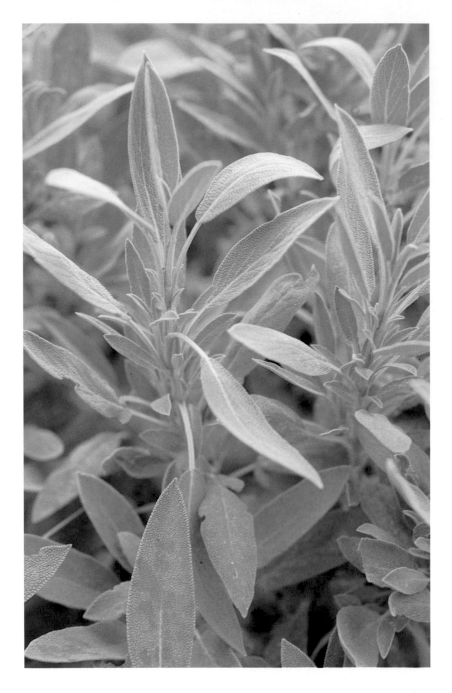

SAGE   *Salvia officinalis*

two hours, otherwise it has no lasting effect. You can make things easier for yourself by using a ready-mixed solution of sage and chamomile extracts. Sage lozenges can also be used between gargling sessions to alleviate pain and discomfort.

One drastic treatment for adults that really separates the "men from the boys" is gargling with undiluted Swedish Bitters. This will bring about fast relief. On our various trips when one of us had a sore throat problem, but no sage tea was available, we were helped out several times by our constant companion, Swedish Bitters (see page 104).

AN HERB FOR LARYNGITIS

Various species of mallow are widely used as decorative garden plants. The wild varieties have beautiful pink blossoms and often thrive close to human dwellings. For medicinal purposes, the leaves and flowers of *Malva neglecta* and *Malva sylvestris* are used. If possible, it is best to harvest them yourself and use them when they are fresh. Then the mucins are most powerful.

Mallow (*Malva neglecta* or *Malva sylvestris*) is a medicinal herb that has curative effects on the mucous membranes of the upper respiratory tract and the oral cavity and throat, because it contains an extraordinary amount of mucin and thus coats and protects inflamed tissues. If you drink pure mallow tea, you will distinctly feel its softening effect in your mouth and throat. We have so often experienced in ourselves and in the case of others how wonderfully this tea helps in cases of laryngitis and pharyngitis! Mallow provides instant relief, especially when these symptoms arise following taxation of the vocal cords. Men and women who are frequently called upon to give long speeches, and singers of every type, should drink mallow tea as a preventative measure. You will achieve the best results with this herb if freshly picked leaves and flowers are used. However, as they are available only from May to November, the dried herb may also be used. In either case, care should be taken in preparing the tea that *boiling water is not used, but rather the flowers and leaves are extracted in lukewarm water overnight,* so that the beneficial plant mucins are preserved.

The anti-inflammatory effect extends itself also to the mucous membranes of the gastrointestinal tract (for an accompanying therapy

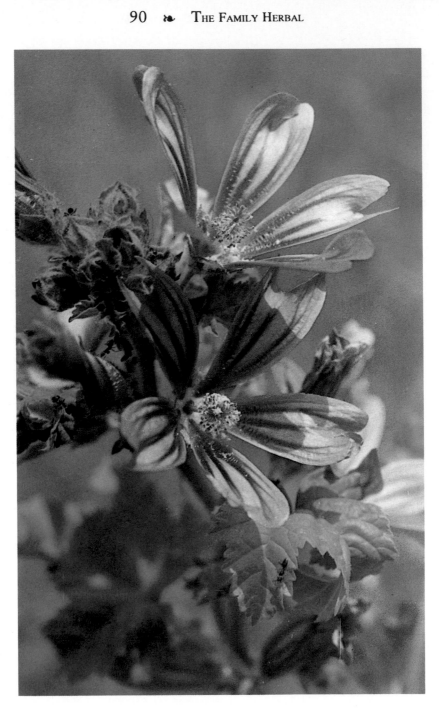

MALLOW   *Malva silvestris*

for gastritis, enteritis, and stomach as well as duodenal ulcers, see also page 160). Even a stubborn case of constipation can be resolved by mallow. In addition, wound-healing properties are attributed to this beautiful flower.

TREATING EARACHE WITH SWEDISH BITTERS

Earache, which often occurs when a cold is in full swing, can be attributed, in most cases, to infection of the middle ear (otitis media). Strangely enough, you usually don't feel it until you are lying quietly in bed trying to go to sleep or you are awakened in the middle of the night by that cutting pain in your ear. The pain can be so excruciating that little children with middle-ear infections cry out and babies constantly toss their heads back and forth. In treating such symptoms we have achieved extraordinary results by applying Swedish Bitters compresses to the affected ear.

During the first nighttime emergency of this type, we weren't so certain our good old Swedish Bitters would be able to help. However, we didn't have any more suitable remedy at hand (such things always happen when you're traveling, staying in a hotel, or camping), so there was nothing to do but try it out. The success of this simple treatment with Swedish Bitters compress was quite evident by next morning. Although the infection was not completely eliminated, the acute pain had become just an unpleasant memory. (See pages 105–107.)

OTHER COMPRESSES FOR EARACHE

The traditional folk remedy for middle-ear infection is the "onion bag," that is, the application of finely chopped onion directly to the ear in the form of a compress. A compress of boiled, mashed potato can also be used. Both of these compresses are surprisingly effective, yet difficult to prepare and a bit awkward to use. The Swedish Bitters compress is much more convenient, so we prefer it.

For further treatment, we recommend repeating the compress procedure overnight for a few nights. During the day, it is advisable to apply a few drops of St. Johnswort oil into the ear canal. In any case, the infection must be cured from the inside by way of echinacea drops, medicinal baths, and the other general defense-improving measures we recommend to fight a cold. Earache should not be taken lightly. Herbal remedies are extremely helpful; however, a physician specializing in natural healing should be consulted who at least monitors the patient's progress, making sure the infection recedes and no complications arise.

More Benefits of Curing a Cold Naturally

Our experience has been that by use of the methods discussed in this and the preceding chapter, a cold can be "intercepted" completely in the beginning or, if it has already taken hold, can be overcome within three days without your having to take to your bed. To be sure, we have observed that patients who take antibiotics require three days to recover as well. The difference is that the antibiotic patients complete their "cold" with depleted resources, a weakened system, and depleted bacterial flora and are left with the job of ridding themselves of many unwanted toxins and chemical residues. Using herbs to "fight" a cold strengthens the entire organism and works without leaving any residue of unwanted chemicals or lingering side effects. By using herbs in this manner, you bring yourself into a closer relationship with your body as you work creatively with natural forces to bring about health and happiness.

∾ 8 ∾

THE EXTRAORDINARY
ELIXIR: SWEDISH BITTERS

*Science is right in what it says; yet it is wrong in
what it leaves unspoken.*
Carl Friedrich von Weizsäcker

Nature has given us the ability to distinguish between four distinctly different tastes: sweet, sour, salty, and bitter. To do so we use the taste buds located over the surface of the tongue, which is divided into four separate taste zones. For example, sweet things are tasted only with the tip of the tongue and bitter things only at the base. And our sense of smell is intimately connected with this sense of taste.

Too Salty, Too Sweet, Too Little Bitter

A review of our daily diet will reveal that most modern Westerners consume sweet, salty, and sour foods every day but hardly ever eat anything bitter. Indeed, we seem to have eliminated bitter tastes from the diet and substituted sweet tastes instead.

This development is very important in regard to Western cultural history. For example, we recently heard of a report about life in China some hundreds of years ago that describes how uncouth and indecent it was to eat sugar and how especially reprehensible this practice was in

93

public! The consequences of eating sugar, according to the author, were moral decay, turning soft, decadence, and loss of strength. By contrast, bitter foods were said to make one strong and courageous. When we consider that sugar in the twentieth century has become an actual addiction, it seems well worth taking a closer look at the consequences of such "abuse." It is an established fact that certain nutritional habits that extend over several generations have a decisive impact on the physical and psychological constitution and character of a nation.

Each of us has a favorite dish that we find piquant—that is, salty—as well as a sweet dessert we adore. But what is your favorite bitter dish or food? In our diet today, there are no more than a few delicately bitter-tasting vegetables—watercress, dandelion, chicory, arugula, and radicchio. Even the almond, which originally tasted quite bitter, has been cultivated and crossbred until it now tastes sweet.

In the typical American diet there is a virtual lack of any bitter-tasting foods. In fact, refined and processed foods, which make up a principal part of the American diet, have reduced the taste spectrum down to virtually two categories: sweet and salty. Our health has suffered in the process, because more and more people have become addicted to salt as well as to sugar.

THE TRADITION OF TAKING "BITTERS"

A bitter taste was once an integral part of the diet of many traditional peoples. The Native Americans ate a great variety of extremely bitter roots whose taste was so harsh and hot that we modern people could not even digest them, much less enjoy them; they would act in our digestive systems like poison. Yet metabolic disorders were practically unknown to primitive and traditional people.

The traditional "spring cure" in Europe, during which bitter and acrid herbs such as dandelion and wild garlic are eaten, is reminiscent of former customs of taste. Even today in France, a rich meal is topped off with an after-dinner "digestive" drink made of bitter herbs, most of which contain calamus root. In the same vein, a wealth of bitter herbs, elixirs, and tonics have been preserved in European medicine up to this very day. Such herbal medicines are extremely important for our health, because they make it possible for our metabolism to reestablish its equilibrium. And a lack of bitter-taste stimuli results in our metabolism becoming unbalanced.

BITTERS FOR LIVER STIMULATION

A naturopathic principle is that bitter substances generally act on the liver. This relationship is seen to correspond to the fact that the liver produces bile, an extremely bitter fluid. When you vomit, but the feeling of nausea still does not pass and you experience the "dry heaves" (there is nothing left for the stomach to discharge), you begin throwing up bile. Anyone who has gone through this awful process knows just how bitter this green liquid tastes. In Chinese medicine, the bitter taste is associated with the liver, just as it is in medical astrology, which formed an integral part of the art and science of early European physicians and alchemists.

The Liver's Vital Role

We can only hint at how vitally important the functioning of the liver is for our health. As physiology teaches us, what the liver does can be divided into two entirely different functions. First, the liver is one of the important exocrine glands of the body, producing the digestive juice bile. This liquid is then conveyed via a system of ducts within the liver to the gallbladder. There it is collected, stored, and released into the small intestine as needed. In the intestine, bile is responsible for breaking down the fats contained in our food, emulsifying and preparing them for absorption.

The second part of the liver's function is complicated and greatly varied. One of its most important roles is the storing of glycogen (blood sugar), the releasing of finely dosed amounts of glycogen into the bloodstream as energy fuel, and the storage of copper, iron, and other trace minerals, as well as the building up of substances for the formation of blood cells, the usage and storage of fats for the production and storage of proteins, and the breaking down of toxins that are dangerous to the body. Environmental toxins of all sorts—heavy metals, chemicals, and pesticides in our food and drinking water, synthetic drugs and medicines—must be dealt with by the liver. To put it in a nutshell, the liver is the central metabolic laboratory for our body. Our lives are absolutely dependent upon our liver functioning in an optimal manner, and our liver in turn depends upon bitter substances for its optimum functioning.

THE REMARKABLE SWEDISH BITTERS HERBAL ELIXIR

Swedish Bitters, an herbal elixir once widely known to activate the liver as well as all the other digestive organs in a very harmonious fashion, has today returned to favor. We owe this welcome development primarily to Maria Treben, who made the elixir well known again through her books *Health from God's Pharmacy* and *Health from God's Garden,* as well as through many lectures in which she enthusiastically reported her success with this remarkable formula.

THE HISTORY OF SWEDISH BITTERS

If you trace the Swedish Bitters formula back through the history of pharmacy, you will find that variations of this same herbal theme have existed over hundreds of years. The elixir has repeatedly appeared in pharmacopeias since the Middle Ages under a variety of names: Hiera picra composita, Tinctura aloes composita, and Species ad longam vitam ("medicine for a long life"). Paracelsus, the great reformer of medicine at the beginning of the sixteenth century, developed the formula of an "Elixir ad longam vitam" containing as its main ingredients aloe, myrrh, and saffron. Since then the various ingredients have no longer been administered in the form of a paste but have been processed into an elixir extracted in alcohol.

In the eighteenth century, a Swedish physician by the name of Samst was said to have discovered the formula from an old family tradition and recorded it anew. Dr. Samst was reported to have lived to the age of 104, when he died—not of old age, but rather as a result of a riding accident! The name Swedish Bitters is attributed to him. A manuscript on Swedish Bitters describing its various uses through forty-three "applications" (i.e., the number of afflictions for which this one single formula can bring relief!) was also compiled by Dr. Samst. Two hundred fifty years later this manuscript found its way into the hands of Maria Treben. Her own recovery from a life-threatening case of typhoid fever through the use of Swedish Bitters marked a turning point in her life and caused her to become deeply committed to herbal medicine.

THE COMPOSITION OF SWEDISH BITTERS

The characteristic feature of all of these formulas, including the present Swedish Bitters elixir (which is composed of eleven herbs and substances), is the masterly way in which the ingredients are combined. For here the principle of synergy applies, that is, that the whole is greater than the sum of its individual parts, which means that the final elixir has a far greater effect than does the taking of each substance separately. In fact, the art of plant-based medicines lies in combining substances that are mutually beneficial and enhance one another. In the Swedish Bitters formula the composition of active ingredients has changed and matured over a period covering a couple of hundred years.

Angelica

One of the most important ingredients in the formula for Swedish Bitters is angelica root (*Angelica archangelica*). The angelica root, or longwort (as this plant is also called), belongs to the group of so-called Amara aromatica, those bitter herbs that contain essential oils as well as bitter ingredients. All herbs of this group, and angelica in particular, stimulate the appetite by increasing the production and secretion of gastric juices, pancreatic juices, and bile.

Botanically speaking, angelica belongs to the family Umbelliferae, a seemingly endless group of species that can at times look so similar that they are very difficult to distinguish one from another. Cases have even been reported in which angelica, which can grow to six or seven feet, has been confused with the extremely dangerous poison hemlock! This is why we urge you not to attempt to collect angelica yourself from the wild unless you possess real botanical expertise. It should also be noted that digging up the root is usually strenuous and tedious work, and even more tedious is the process of drying and additional preparation. Moreover, long-term storage of angelica root causes other problems due to its strong aroma, which attracts more insects than any other herb. For these reasons, digging angelica root yourself makes sense only in areas where the herb grows in great abundance (which is sadly no longer the case in Germany) and for those passionate herbalists who love the strong, acrid taste of the fresh root. These adventurous people like to chew a small piece of the root each day for general strength, much as the Chinese chew ginseng (see chapter 16).

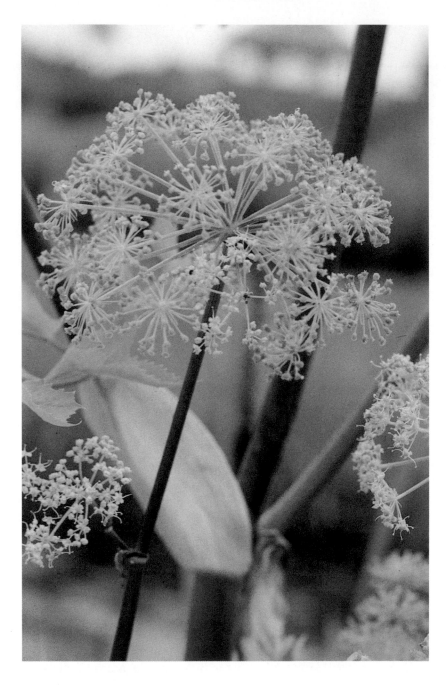

Angelica   *Angelica archangelica*

Angelica is indigenous to Europe and Asia (mainly in the northern-most regions). It grows naturally along rivers and in moist meadows and light forests, and it can thrive in a garden given a shady moist spot, especially quite near a pond. However, the enormous quantities of an-gelica root that are processed by the liquor industry (for after-dinner digestives) require a cultivated source.

Any symptoms of indigestion can be cured with the help of angelica tea or tincture. The root strengthens the stomach, disinfects the intes-tines, alleviates flatulence, and relieves intestinal colic as well. As in the case of all roots, it is best to prepare a cold infusion: pour one cup of cold water over one teaspoon of angelica root, let stand in a saucepan for several hours, then boil for two minutes, steep two more minutes, strain off, and serve.

Angelica is almost always combined with other herbal stomachic and digestive aids in elixirs, tea blends, and herbal tablets. If you want to use angelica root by itself, do so sparingly. It is not recommended for continuous application over a long period of time. A beneficial cure for the digestive organs, which should be undertaken no longer than four weeks, would be one cup of angelica tea three times a day before meals, or twenty drops of angelica tincture three times a day.

Other Ingredients

Besides angelica, Swedish Bitters contains the root of the carline thistle (*Carlina acaulis*), which possesses bacteriostatic properties (that is, in-hibits bacterial growth) and acts on the stomach as well. It also has a diuretic effect. Zedoary root (*Curcuma zedoaria*) is another ingredient that stimulates the secretion of gastric juices and bile.

Rhubarb (*Rheum palmatum*) is another important bitter plant. Its roots are used for treating inflammations of the gastrointestinal tract, and it is a mild laxative as well. Myrrh is the air-dried milky exudate of a tree indigenous to Africa (*Commiphora molmol*). When administered internally, the extract of these resin-containing myrrh granules acts on intestinal infection and flatulence. When used externally, it acts as an astringent and disinfectant. The leaves of the aloe (*Aloe capensis* and *Aloe ferox*) are used to make a thickened juice that stimulates bowel action. The manna ash, or flowering ash (*Fraxinus ornus*), supplies a milky exudate that is air-dried. Its sap is obtained by tapping the tree, much as the North American maple is tapped. Manna is a very mild laxative, well tolerated even by small children and babies. It reduces the resorption of liquid in the small intestine and thus stimulates peristalsis (the wormlike movement of the colon that propels its contents along the intestinal tract).

Senna leaves (*Senna angustifolia, Senna acutifolia*) is a further ingredient of Swedish Bitters with a laxative action. Yet the effect of the laxative ingredients is on the whole relatively weak, because of the way in which the mixture is made. Saffron (*Crocus sativus*) is most familiar to people as a spice. It is extremely expensive, because only a tiny part of the plant's flower is used—the brick-red stigmas or female organs of the plant, which must be picked by hand. (Thirty-five to forty thousand flower blossoms are required to obtain a single pound of this most precious of all herbs.) Saffron is also a medicinal substance that has a soothing and antispasmodic effect on the stomach and is even capable of sedating the stomach nerves.

Another component found in Swedish Bitters is theriac (*Electuarium theriacale*). This in itself is a powerful herbal mixture with a long-revered tradition, composed of seven different medicinal herbs and spices: angelica root, cimicifuga root, valerian root, cinnamon bark, zedoary root, cardamom, and myrrh. Finally, Swedish Bitters contains camphor, which like manna is obtained from the trunk of a tree (*Cinnamomum camphora*); camphor stimulates blood circulation. Swedish Bitters elixir is made by extracting all the herbs together for several days in high-proof alcohol and then diluting the elixir to its proper strength.

PREPARING SWEDISH BITTERS ELIXIR YOURSELF

Many people enjoy making their own Swedish Bitters elixir from dried herbs. A 3.15-ounce (90 gram) packet of premixed "Swedish Bitters" herbs is available commercially, according to the following recipe:

> 3½ *parts manna*
> 2 *parts aloe*
> 2 *parts rhubarb root*
> 2 *parts senna leaves*
> 2 *parts theriac venezian*
> 2 *parts zedoary root*
> 1 *part angelica root*

1 *part carline thistle root*
1 *part myrrh*
½ *part camphor*
½ *part saffron*

Place the herbs in a clean, clear glass bottle and pour 50 fluid ounces of 80 proof spirits (40 percent alcohol by volume) over the herbs. You can use brandy, vodka, or any good quality fruit spirits. Let the preparation stand for fourteen days, shaking the contents daily. Filter through a large kitchen strainer lined with cheesecloth and store in a dark-tinted glass bottle. This homemade mixture tends to be quite strong and not as smooth as the professionally made Swedish Bitters elixir. Most people prefer to use it only for external applications.

USING SWEDISH BITTERS INTERNALLY

Experience has shown that the Swedish Bitters elixir has a remarkably wide range of applications. First and foremost, it is traditionally acknowledged as an effective substance for "purifying the blood." "Blood purification" may be defined as a process that frees the body of superfluous metabolic substances and waste products by acting on the metabolism of the entire organism in fluids, tissues, and cells, and simultaneously stimulates the major excretory organs, the kidneys, liver, and intestines. The herbs that were said by folk medicine to purify the blood correspond exactly to this spectrum of effects. The protagonist of this wide range of actions is the Swedish Bitters elixir.

It was not by accident that Swedish Bitters began its new career as a self-medication that people used because they felt good about it and believed in its value—and not as a medicine prescribed by a physician. Practice has shown that a blood-cleansing treatment with Swedish Bitters can considerably reduce fatigue, listlessness, and a run-down feeling over time. For rheumatic pain, as a stimulation therapy for allergies, and for generally cleaning out the body, we recommend a course of treatment extending over eight to ten weeks, twice a year.

Blood purification is intended as a preventative measure, whereas afflictions of the digestive tract necessitate concrete and perceptible relief from an entire range of symptoms: bloated feeling, flatulence, pressure pains, stomach cramps, constipation, indigestion when eating certain rich or fatty foods, nausea, heartburn, lack of appetite, and occasional bouts with severe headaches after meals. All of the digestive organs are involved when symptoms of this type occur, because the functions of the stomach, liver, gallbladder, pancreas, and small and large intestines are so closely associated with one another. The affliction or failure of any one of these digestive organs will result in disturbances for all the others as well. Depending upon the patient's diet, the symptoms listed here occur with changing frequency, intensity, and dominance, since the organs are not able to work together as they should. What then occurs is both a quantitative and qualitative deficiency and an imbalance of the digestive enzymes. Psychological tension and stress also play a major role and are more often the trigger of such symptoms in women than they are in men.

We have seen clinical studies conducted (double-blind tests) involving the treatment of indigestion with Swedish Bitters Elixir. These studies have indicated conclusively that dyspepsia, accompanied by the symptoms described above, can be improved by administering the elixir, and that Swedish Bitters is quite well tolerated. The proper dosage is two teaspoons three times a day, before meals. If you normally do not suffer from indigestion but on occasion have an extra-rich, heavy meal, then it is advisable to take two teaspoons after eating.

Swedish Bitters is indispensable for us when we're traveling. When we are invited for large heavy meals (mostly late at night) or try out foods we have never tasted before or are simply not accustomed to, we truly need our Swedish Bitters! A swallow of it guarantees that in spite of the food we will get a peaceful night's rest and awaken refreshed in the morning.

Swedish Bitters does credit to its name, for it is really quite bitter. According to the guidelines of the German Pharmacopeia, it has a bitter rating of 1,000. By comparison, freshly squeezed artichoke juice has a rating of merely 30! Thus, we advise you to dilute Swedish Bitters in a cup of herbal tea, water, or juice. Here's a tip: one glass of orange juice with two teaspoons of Swedish Bitters tastes just like a specialty drink currently in vogue in Europe, known as a Campari Orange.

A great deal is known about the acting mechanisms of bitter herbs based on the wide range of scientific investigations that have been carried out. Although it was believed for a long time that the increased secretion of saliva and gastric juices provided by bitter herbal ingredients was only possible via the stimulation of the autonomic nervous system, it is now known that the gastric mucosa itself is stimulated on contact with bitter substances to increase production of gastric acids. This sets up a chain reaction whose immediate result is improved food utilization and absorption. The elucidation of this reactive mechanism is of importance in that it answers the question whether or not you have to taste bitters for them to do you any good or whether they are still effective when taken in the form of a capsule. The answer is yes, bitter substances work even if you do not taste them.

Therefore, for those who cannot get accustomed to the bitter taste of the elixir, there is the alternative of using Swedish Bitters capsules. This option gives you the benefits of balancing your diet and stimulating your liver and digestion without having to be subjected to the bitter taste. However, we tend to think that the effect is stronger with the liquid elixir, since it works both by direct stimulation and by nerve stimulation. For anyone who has a problem with the alcohol in Swedish Bitters liquid elixir, capsules are the solution, because they contain no alcohol. In this context, please refer to our general discussion of the use of alcohol as a base in natural medications in chapter 4 (pages 39–40).

Regarding the general vitalizing and strengthening effect of bitter herbs, please refer to page 166. In addition, over many years we have collected numerous indications and hints about a general improvement of the immune system through bitters, which is the subject of some new clinical studies recently begun.

One condition where the internal application of Swedish Bitters would be detrimental is diarrhea. If it has already been used, discontinue it, as the problem will be worsened. Individuals with sensitive digestive systems or who are susceptible to bouts of diarrhea should be very careful not to take too great a dose. In such cases, one-half teaspoon per day may be best. *Swedish Bitters elixir is also not allowed in cases of intestinal obstruction (ileus) or during pregnancy and breastfeeding.*

SWEDISH BITTERS EXTERNALLY

In addition, Swedish Bitters can be administered externally, a process with which we have personally had phenomenal success. *When administered externally it is always used undiluted.* Swedish Bitters is a boon any time local infections need to be treated; it can be either dabbed on like a lotion or applied in the form of a compress. To disinfect and soothe insect bites, for example, simply apply some elixir directly to the skin on the affected area. The elixir can also be dabbed onto fever sores on the lips or discharging pimples, which causes them to recede very quickly, sometimes within only a few hours. Similarly, when Swedish Bitters is applied to chicken pox blisters they crust over and begin to heal quite quickly. We have seen this happen not only with our own children but also with the children of many friends. Chicken pox blisters usually take three days from the time they appear as red spots to develop, grow to full bloom, fill with fluid, and then fade away. When patients, on our advice, dabbed Swedish Bitters on the evolving red eruptions several times a day, this cycle took only a single day!

In chapter 7 (page 89) we described how Swedish Bitters can be used for gargling in cases of throat infections and hoarseness. Three tablespoons diluted in a glass of water does the trick nicely. If you're hardy enough (or even enjoy the taste, as a growing number of people do) to gargle with Swedish Bitters undiluted, you can expect the infection to recede even more quickly.

In chapter 10, where we will discuss headache, we mention that one of the many possible causes of this condition can be eye strain. If you suffer occasionally from such a condition, try to lie down for ten minutes (even at work) and place two cotton balls moistened with Swedish Bitters on the closed eyelids. Press them down gently and you will feel a delightfully soothing, cooling effect. (To avoid stinging the eyes, be sure to keep the eyelids closed, and rinse them with clear water before opening them.)

THE SWEDISH BITTERS COMPRESS

In our family, the Swedish Bitters compress has literally become a universal remedy. For example, we remember clearly the case of our daughter Sarah, who stepped on a bee while playing beside a pool in California when she was five years old. We immediately grabbed our bottle of Swedish Bitters and applied plenty of the elixir to the skin around the sting. We applied a cotton swab soaked in Swedish Bitters as a small compress directly to the wound, and Sarah felt relief almost immediately. If we had not seen it ourselves, we would never have believed that Swedish Bitters could work so rapidly! After ten to fifteen minutes there

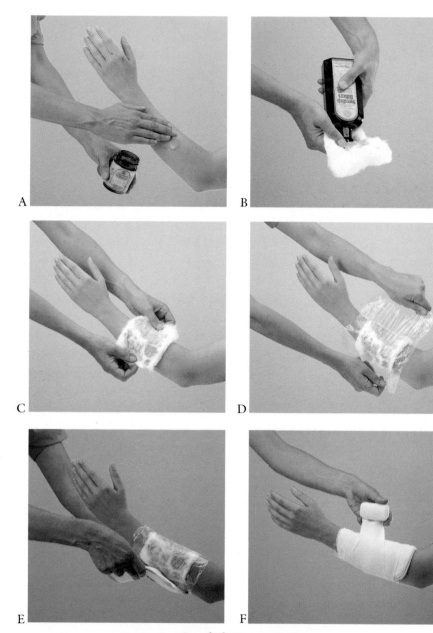

FIGURE 8. *Swedish Bitters Compress*

A. Apply a thick layer of calendula ointment to the skin of the affected area.

B. Moisten a piece of cotton cloth (the size
of the area to be treated) with the elixir.

C. Place the moist cotton on the skin.

D. Cover with a piece of plastic wrap

slightly larger than the compress on all
sides.

E. Cover with a woolen or flannel cloth or
a hand towel.

F. Secure the compress in place with a
scarf or cloth bandage.

was hardly any more swelling and no more pain. In the case of insect bites and stings we have observed that it is often crucial to apply the elixir as quickly as possible. In Malaysia, we once met two ladies who reported the amazing story that one of them had actually saved the life of her daughter, who had been stung repeatedly by huge tropical hornets, by immediately applying Swedish Bitters!

The throat compress for infected tonsils and a compress for infections of the middle ear were described in chapter 7 (pages 86–87 and 91). A Swedish Bitters compress can also help heal slow-healing injuries and infected wounds that throb and hurt. The general anti-inflammatory effect of the Swedish Bitters compress has also proved successful in connection with rheumatic (arthritic) pain and for bringing relief in acute asthmatic conditions. When one of our children complains of a stomachache, the first thing we do is to directly apply a Swedish Bitters compress overnight. As a rule, the child feels much better the next morning. Someone who complains of a headache should lie down for fifteen minutes and apply a washcloth soaked with Swedish Bitters and squeezed out carefully to the forehead or the back of the head and the neck. When administered externally, Swedish Bitters stimulates the blood circulation and is thus able to relax constricted blood vessels, as in the case of migraine. (See also pages 129–133.)

How to Make a Swedish Bitters Compress

First, some important points. When administered externally, the elixir is never diluted. However, extended exposure to the elixir will cause the skin to dry out because of the high alcohol content, and it is therefore necessary to protect the skin. (This does not apply to the simple dabbing on of Swedish Bitters for minor problems such as insect bites or blemishes.) This is why when using Swedish Bitters as a compress, calendula ointment should be applied to the skin area that is to be covered (see page 227). This rich, fatty ointment will prevent the skin from being damaged, even when the compress is left on for many hours.

To make the compress, a piece of absorbent cotton cloth the size of the area to be treated is wetted with the Swedish Bitters elixir; it should only be moistened, not dripping wet. The moist, cool piece of cotton is now placed on the skin (which has been prepared with calendula cream), then covered with a piece of ordinary plastic kitchen wrap trimmed a little larger than the compress itself. The entire compress is then covered with a woolen or flannel cloth or small towel and secured by wrapping a scarf or cloth bandage around it (see figure 8). The compress should be left on for at least an hour. In most cases it is advisable to leave it on overnight, as it causes the least inconvenience when the patient is asleep.

Please note that the dark brown liquid elixir leaves pronounced stains, which is one of the reasons the plastic wrap must be used to protect clothing or bedding. If stains do occur, a normal washing will remove them from the fabric. For easy application, especially when large areas of the body are to be treated, use a disposable diaper. A disposable diaper consists of a soft, absorbent cellulose layer welded to a thin plastic covering that serves as a moisture barrier. Thus when a disposable diaper is used for applying the elixir, kitchen wrap need not be used.

When used externally, Swedish Bitters elixir has a cooling, anti-inflammatory, disinfecting, and contracting effect and promotes local circulation. From a pharmacological point of view, this can be attributed to the camphor and myrrh it contains. However, this alone does not completely explain its comprehensive effect when it is administered externally.

SWEDISH BITTERS STORIES

We have received a great variety of testimonials from all over the world about Swedish Bitters, including strange and unusual reports according to which people, horses, cats, and dogs have been cured of a myriad of serious afflictions. One of the most curious stories came from the United States and told of a pet white rat who was dying from some poison that it had eaten. After a dose of Swedish Bitters it recovered within a single day and was again in the pink of health, we assume running through its cage in search of cheese.

From near our hometown in Germany, a farmer told us about his sick cow: the animal had taken ill and had not moved for days. A veterinarian was called, but he said there was nothing that could be done; the cow must be put away. The farmer's wife suggested that they give it one last try with Swedish Bitters, so they poured a large bottle of the elixir into a pail of water and offered it to the cow. Amazingly enough, she drank it all, and when the farmer and his wife came to check her an hour later the cow was on her feet, swishing her tail happily!

The renaissance of Swedish Bitters Elixir and its acceptance in so many countries all over the world is a phenomenon in itself. In Germany, it is sold through pharmacies as a home remedy. In France and the Netherlands, it is used daily by thousands of people as a revitalizing tonic. In the United States, it is available in more than five thousand natural and health food stores and is recommended by a growing number of herbologists, naturopaths, and chiropractors. Chief Two Trees, a Cherokee medicine man from North Carolina, among many others, recommends it to all his patients. In Malaysia it is a prized possession, and even in remote parts of India it is prescribed by physicians.

9

HEALING HERBS
FOR YOUR NERVOUS SYSTEM

What happens in the body is not what is essential.
This is why the ability to heal demands more than
simple knowledge of the body.

Rolling Thunder, Cherokee healer

Now, more than ever before, we need natural alternatives to the six million chemical tranquilizers taken every year in the United States (consumption of which has doubled in the past ten years). These capsules and pills cannot be employed indefinitely to combat the effects of daily stress and "nerves," nor can the powerful synthetic drugs they contain provide the proper rest our bodies need. Perhaps here more dangerously than in any other situation, we have focused on combating the symptoms while ignoring the cause; today, no one can deny that we have arrived at a cul-de-sac in our irresponsible misuse of narcotics.

Thankfully, phytotherapy has an answer to these problems. Stress, nervousness, overstimulation, and insomnia are symptoms that usually occur together, and it is more obvious in these instances than it is in the case of other manifestations of disease that they are emotional and mental in origin.

WHAT IS DISEASE?

Perhaps our attitude toward disease is already apparent from the preceding chapters. We are of the opinion that every disorder, without exception, has a uniquely personal origin. After many years of experience with a variety of sensitive methods of treatment (such as breathing therapy, yoga, and subtle forms of massage), we have learned that every negative emotion, every irritation, in fact all uneasiness, has a "mirror" physical effect in the form of resistance, tension, or rigidity, even though these effects are at times barely noticeable. The more constantly the person is plagued by ill-feeling, a sense of inferiority, anxiety, or discord, the more his or her body falls prey to these tensions. Eventually these result in an energy deficit in a particular organ or system of organs and manifest as what we call "functional disturbances," which in turn ultimately lead to "organic disorders."

It is actually of little importance whether the energy imbalance is expressed as gastric ulcers, diabetes, diminished resistance, high blood pressure, gout attacks, sleeplessness, or cancer. The fact is that each one of us creates his or her own diseases, and in the end it is only the individual who can effect a cure. It is no accident that the words *whole, holy,* and *heal* stem from the same root. Our final aim can only be to make ourselves whole and healthy.

Nervous Complaints

The young, the old, and the middle-aged all suffer from nervous complaints to the same extent; babies and infants are no exception. Take, for example, the young person who feels unrecognized by his or her peers and reacts by being restless and nervous; the father who feels constantly bogged down at work and suffers from severe, recurring headaches; the single mother who is so worried about her financial circumstances that she loses her appetite and can hardly swallow the meals she so desperately needs; the grandfather who is unreasonably annoyed by the neighbor's dog and suffers regularly from a nervous heart complaint; the child who feels dreadful pressure at school to get good grades and has problems falling asleep the night before a big exam; and the baby that feels unwanted and uncared-for and constantly cries itself to sleep. They can all find natural help and alleviation of their unwanted symptoms through the use of herbs that calm, relax, and relieve. The most important of these herbs are balm, St. Johnswort, and valerian. To these we would add hops, passion flowers (maypops), oats, and lavender.

BALM

Balm (*Melissa officinalis*) is not just an effective medicinal but also a pleasantly fragrant and delightful-tasting herb. Because of its fragrance, it is also known as lemon balm. It does not grow wild but is easily cultivated as a garden plant in good, well-nourished soil receiving plenty of sunlight. If you are harvesting the leaves yourself, it is important to pick them before the plant goes to flower since their fragrance changes afterward. Balm attracts bees in swarms, and fresh balm leaves are a delicious flavoring herb in salads, sauces, soups, and vegetable dishes. This versatile herb would earn its place in our garden on this account alone. It is the leaves that are used medicinally, as they contain the essential oils, as well as tannins, bitters, and flavonoids.

Balm Tea

Balm is employed in the form of a tea, as a tincture, and for adding to baths. The tea is a great help in cases of "nerves" and nervous sleeplessness. Note that this herb represents an exception to normal tea-making procedure and should be dosed higher than usual: three teaspoonsful of balm leaves should be used per cup. Here it is particularly important to cover the pot or cup while the tea steeps for five minutes and afterward to return the condensed drops of liquid from the underside of the cover back to the tea, for the sedative and spasmolytic (spasm-relieving) effect of balm is mainly caused by its essential oils, which are extracted immediately upon brewing and evaporate easily.

Balm tea is particularly effective when stress has affected the stomach and the digestive organs. It loosens the feeling of tightness in the stomach and dissolves the cramplike pains that sometimes occur, and it also stimulates the appetite. For such complaints, one to two cups of balm tea should be taken every day. In the case of children, one cup before bed often suffices to transform nervousness and worry about "that test tomorrow" into pleasant, confident dreams. Balm leaves combine well with other soothing herbs, which is why they always find their way into every "goodnight" tea.

Jonas's Story

Our son, Jonas, experienced a phase in his school career when he was very upset with his bad grades. He felt a great deal of pressure, con-

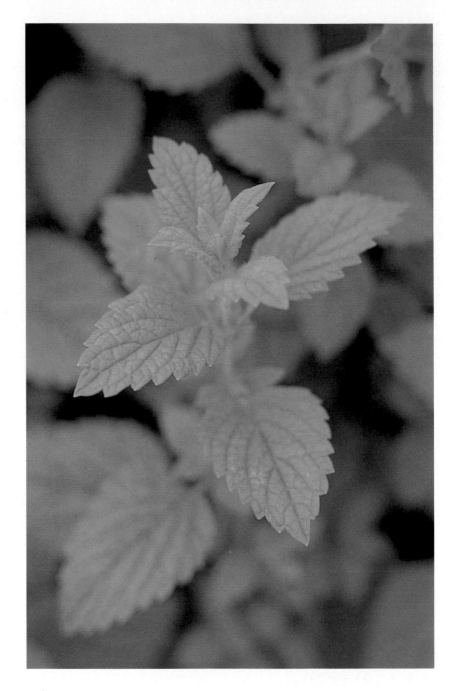

BALM   *Melissa officinalis*

stantly had a worried look on his face, became extremely nervous, lost his appetite, and could not fall asleep at night. We tried our best to take this in stride and viewed his condition as simply one of his first "puberty crises." After some weeks filled with many talks with Jonas and his teachers, we were worried enough about his worrying to place him on a tea cure with balm leaves and St. Johnswort. He had to drink several cups of tea made from these two herbs every day, especially in the evening and at dinnertime. After about two weeks we could see a distinct improvement in his condition: he was sleeping normally, and the "crisis" feelings were fading away. Ever since that time he has known that "his" tea mixture will help him when he feels worried or overly nervous about the next day at school.

Balm Tincture and Bath

Balm tincture is used for more or less the same indications as is balm tea with a little more emphasis on the "nervous stomach" and digestive organs reacting to tension and stress. As with any tincture, of course, it is appropriate to administer when traveling or at any place or time where or when it is not possible to prepare the tea.

Never underestimate the effectiveness of a balm full bath. Anyone who can do so should enjoy this superbly relaxing experience two to three times a week before going to bed. Even if you do not suffer from the symptoms mentioned above but merely wish to recover after a particularly trying day's work or a long drive, a balm bath is a welcome gift. It is a real help with small children who get overactive or fidgety and who often get a bit crazy when they are overtired.

VALERIAN

Valerian (*Valeriana officinalis*) has an even stronger sedative effect than balm. It enables you to relax both physically and mentally when you are overworked or experiencing tension and stress, without making you tired, creating a narcotized sensation, or causing dependency as is usual with chemical psychotherapeutics. People who easily become irritated or overexcited can use valerian during the day as a gentle sedative as often as they like without detrimental side effects.

The name *valerian* is derived from the Latin *valere* ("to be well, be worth, be strong"), which gives testimony to the high esteem in which valerian was held in ancient times, as does its English folk name, "all-heal." Valerian grows tall with feathery leaves and whitish or pale pink flowers and thrives preferably in wet meadows close to streams and in clearings of deciduous forests. German folk names such as *Mondwurzel* ("moon root") and *Undinenkraut* ("Undine's herb") reflect the preference of this herb for a watery environment as well. Valerian can be grown in the family garden, and the roots can be cultivated in the second or third year. Many gardeners claim that planting valerian among other vegetables helps all the plants in the garden to grow well.

The smell of valerian root (known in Germany as *Katzenkraut,* or "cat's herb") seems to totally fascinate and even hypnotize cats, so if you have a cat in your house you should be careful how you handle and store this herb. If you spill a drop of tea or tincture on the counter, your cat will be attracted to that spot and will sit on it, mesmerized, for a long time.

Valerian tea is rather neglected nowadays as a homemade remedy because the roots smell so strongly during preparation and the smell lingers about in the house. The flavor is also quite "singular," so you should always use valerian in a mixture with other pleasant-tasting herbs, as in the following recipe.

❧ Nerve-Calming Tea ❧

8 parts valerian root
6 parts hops
3 parts peppermint leaves
3 parts hibiscus flowers

It is best to soak these herbs overnight in lukewarm water, heat up to drinking temperature in the morning, and then strain them off. The results are excellent, particularly for older people who often need calming on account of a nervous heart. The special thing about valerian is that it is so calming and relaxing, yet it does not inhibit concentration and awareness. Can the same be said about any chemical tranquilizer?

Valerian Tincture

Today, tincture of valerian is quite popular again. It can be purchased readymade and is very easy to use. Our grandmothers used to keep it at the ready in their handbags, for in the "good old days" a European lady might fall into a swoon at any moment and therefore always carried a little bottle of valerian tincture to avoid being embarrassed.

The proper dose for valerian tincture to combat sleeplessness is one teaspoonful in half a glass of water before going to bed. A suitable dose for nervous heart complaints is thirty drops, three times daily. Valerian tincture is absolutely safe and can be taken as needed anytime throughout the day whenever a calming effect is desired.

A pleasant tasting, calming tea blend suitable for the whole family after the evening meal or as a nightcap is the following.

❧ Goodnight Tea ❧

4 parts St. Johnswort
3 parts balm leaves
2 parts valerian root
2 parts cowslip flowers
2 parts hawthorn leaves and flowers
2 parts passion flower (Maypops)
2 parts oats (straw)
2 parts hops
1 part lavender blossoms

Hop Cones

Hop cones (*Humulus lupulus*) not only are essential for brewing beer but are pharmacologically accepted as a sedative by both folk medicine and modern science and hence are recommended for nerves and sleeplessness. A mixture of balm, hops, and passion flower has proved of value for children having difficulties at school, for autonomic nervous disorder, and for menopausal symptoms. The simple formula is as follows.

❧ Calming Tea ❧

8 parts balm leaves
6 parts hops
6 parts passion flower

HERBAL SLEEPING PILLOWS

The herbal sleeping pillow is a tradition of long standing. In these days aromatherapy is again attracting attention, even though it was for a long

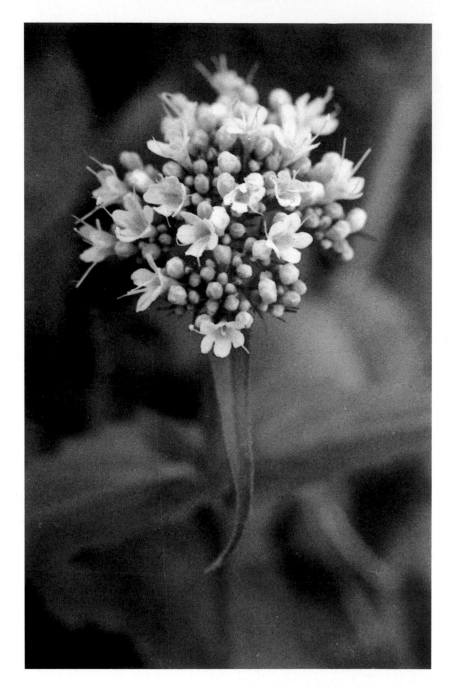

VALERIAN   *Valeriana officinalis*

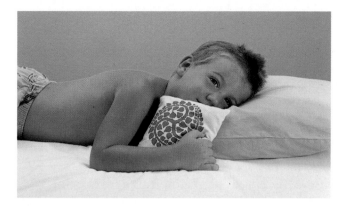

FIGURE 9
Herbal Sleeping Pillow
Place the pillow beside the head and breathe in its scent.

time completely ignored by doctors and scientists. The fact is that the soothing effect of balm leaves, hops, and lavender blossoms depends on their essential oils, and these beneficial substances are best consumed by inhalation. To prepare a really effective herbal pillow, fill a six-inch square cotton bag with balm, hops, lavender, and St. Johnswort. Either lie down with your head directly on the pillow, or place it beside your head while you sleep (see figure 9). In our experience, small children are objectively calmed down and often become so attached to these little comforters that they can't bear to part with them.

Babies who do not want to sleep and who cry a lot are usually suffering from stomachache, teething problems, or some other discomfort. An herbal pillow filled with chamomile and hops placed on the tummy (on top of the clothing) can sometimes work wonders!

Many years ago we created an herbal pillow as a Christmas present for our customers at the Market Pharmacy. A number of the people who received them returned to tell us that the pillow had helped them sleep at last without the need for sleeping pills. This made us so enthusiastic that we introduced the herbal pillow into the product line of our company. Here's what the pillow contains:

❧ Herbal Sleeping Pillow ☙

4 parts melilot
3 parts orange blossom
3 parts chamomile blossoms
3 parts lavender blossoms
3 parts balm leaves
3 parts rose petals

WHY CAN'T WE SLEEP?

Perhaps the success of the herbal sleeping pillow provides an insight into what is really wrong when we find we cannot sleep: we have obviously fixed our minds on something. Our customers, for example, had the fixed idea that they could not get to sleep without sleeping tablets, and they gave up this fixation only when we offered them something "better" to take its place. Many night-duty nurses can report excellent results when placebo sleeping pills are given to patients who feel they need medication. We have fond memories of a humorous conversation with a psychologist friend who amusingly described the reactions of a patient who suffered from chronic insomnia and was very upset about it. Our friend tried to convince his patient of the benefits of staying up all night, simply to stop him from being so angry at himself! All his efforts were to no avail. Whether sleeplessness is chronic or only temporary, we should be aware that we have become excessively fixated on some thought, anxiety, or desire and are just not able to rid ourselves of it.

It is well known that insomnia often has childhood origins. Bed should be a place of absolute security for the infant, and a mother should do everything possible to avoid disturbing factors such as excess noise, light that is too bright, or unfavorable energy from any source. Bedtime should always be made attractive to older children by combining it with something pleasant: reading or telling stories, singing a lullaby, lighting a candle and praying, or gazing at the twinkling magic of the night sky. In this way going to bed is turned into a ritual of enjoyment, and every child will thrive on this special time of undivided parental attention. It is completely wrong to threaten to send a child to bed if he or she misbehaves or neglects to do something. Such threats turn bed and sleep into a punishment—hardly the proper image to associate with such a vital mental and physical human necessity.

Autosuggestion, meditation, and whole-body relaxation are all highly effective methods for combatting insomnia. The practice of deep breathing is the foremost and most simple sedative of all. Children readily learn to enjoy and manage their breath, calming themselves easily, if they are correctly taught.

St. Johnswort

St. Johnswort (*Hypericum perforatum*) is the most important medicinal herb for insomnia and for the nervous system in general, as well as having many other fields of application. It grows in meadows, open woodland, and sunny glades, and its bright yellow flowers bloom around St. John's Day, marking the summer solstice, when the sun is at its northernmost point on the celestial sphere. The Latin term *perforatum* ("punctured") in the plant's scientific name refers to the many tiny black dots that cover the leaves and flowers. These are not in fact holes, as was once thought, but little glands filled with the red dyestuff hypericine. If you harvest St. Johnswort, a sure sign of identification is the red color that dyes your skin as you rub the flower and leaves between your thumb and index finger.

Effect on the Nervous System

St. Johnswort has a clearly sedative effect, which is why we employ it in calming and sleep-bringing teas; but its main property is its ability to fortify the entire nervous system. Recent scientific research has shown that St. Johnswort can be regarded as an herbal antidepressant. Its primary active ingredient, hypericine, acts as a monoamino oxidase inhibitor, much like a "pep pill," but without altering your body's chemistry or deadening the central nervous system. Biochemists have now discovered that hypericine is also a type of plant substance that enables the organism to increase its intake of oxygen on a cellular level (vesicular breathing) and thereby enhances our energy level and overall health significantly. For example, in the case of a cancerous cell in which the basic metabolic intake of oxygen has been inhibited or is nonexistent, when the cell's breathing is restored to normal capacity the cell can be restored to health.

Tea or tincture is the proper form of administration for autonomic nervous disturbances, depressive states, anxiety attacks, and conditions of "nerves." Admittedly, it is necessary to take the tea or tincture several times a day for many weeks, perhaps even months, to achieve good results. But what a godsend this herb is by comparison to the psycho-

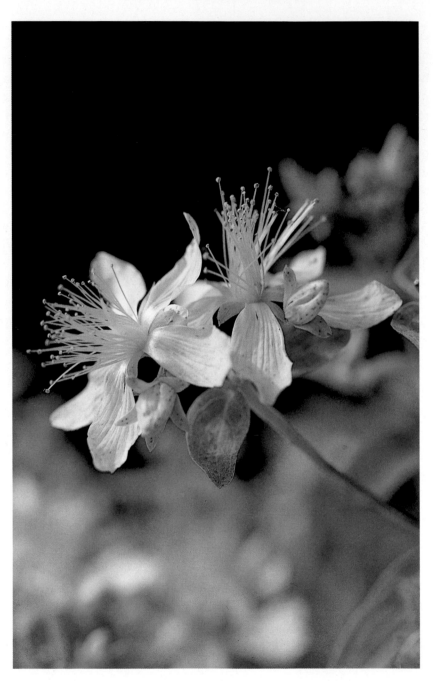

ST. JOHNSWORT *Hypericum perforatum*

pharmaceuticals normally prescribed as antidepressants, which cause severe, debilitating damage to the central nervous system and carry in their wake the diabolical specter of addiction!

A Possible Side Effect

There is one possible side effect that we must bring to your attention: namely, *St. Johnswort increases photosensitivity*. This means that men and women who are sensitive to light—particularly people with fair skin—may react with sunburnlike skin irritation or a sun allergy if they are exposed to strong sunlight during the period of treatment. We ourselves have never heard of a single case of this occurring, but nevertheless the warning needs to be given. If, for example, a patient is in the habit of using a solarium regularly, it would be best to discontinue the practice while taking St. Johnswort.

Uses

Treatment with St. Johnswort is ideal in cases where a person has to adjust to a painful personal loss such as the death of a loved one, separation or divorce, and so on, and therefore has a marked tendency toward depression. It can also be recommended as a tea, together with equal parts of hops and balm, for variations in mood caused by hormonal changes during menopause. (See also pages 209–210.)

Continuous therapy with St. Johnswort also restores zest for life to older people who feel lonely and cast aside. Here it is ideal in combination with balm and hawthorn (see page 141). St. Johnswort tea in combination with balm is also wonderful for children and adults alike who experience problems with concentration. This tea has a wonderful flavor and is therefore an excellent breakfast beverage, especially before starting a demanding day at work or school.

For stressful situations we have created a wonderful tea with St. Johnswort that is very suitable for use as a family and household tea.

🪶 Stress Tea 🪶

6 parts St. Johnswort
6 parts balm leaves
4 parts speedwell
2 parts cowslip flowers
1 part rose hips
1 part raspberry leaves

We have personally observed amazingly good results in children with a quite concentrated tincture of *Hypericum perforatum:* An otherwise very intelligent and clever girl of six years had been suffering off and on from bed-wetting over the course of several years. Also, during the day it often happened that her panties got wet, and her mother—understandably—was very upset about this condition. After she had taken the tincture for two days, the bed-wetting stopped and never came back! This initial success encouraged us to prescribe the tincture more often to children, and subsequently we had similar success with children afflicted by stuttering, extreme fear of darkness, and nervous exhaustion. The dosage for an adult is twenty to thirty drops before meals two to three times per day. Children, depending upon their age and weight, may be given about half this quantity.

Homemade St. Johnswort Oil

Whereas the whole plant is employed in the preparation of teas or tinctures, only the fresh flowers are used to create St. Johnswort oil. Fill a transparent preserve jar or widemouthed bottle with several handfuls of freshly picked flowers, then pour in good quality olive or soy oil until the flowers are covered and close the jar tightly. Allow it to extract for several weeks outdoors or at the window in as much sunlight as possible. When the oil has become dark red in color (after two to six weeks), strain off the flowers, then squeeze them to get the rest of the oil out. It is remarkable that the dark red coloration, which is a sign of the extraction of the hypericine, takes place only under the direct influence of sunlight; this factor serves as a further indication of the plant's strong relationship with the sun.

External Applications

St. Johnswort oil has a pronounced healing effect on mild burns and sunburns (first and second degree). When applied externally, it has proved its worth as a treatment for dermatoses such as chronic eczema and other vesicular skin diseases, especially those that react positively to exposure to the sun. In this context, it makes sense that St. Johnswort can, on the one hand, cause irritation in light-sensitive people and, on the other hand, alleviate depressions, which are known to occur more frequently in dull, cloudy weather and in seasons and places where little sun shines. It is as though St. Johnswort were in some way a carrier and provider of sunlight.

St. Johnswort Oil Compress

St. Johnswort oil is also employed for healing cuts and scrapes. We have had excellent results from compresses of warm St. Johnswort oil in cases of chronic muscle stiffness; tense, knotted muscles; sciatica; and lumbago. Such applications can provide relief as well in cases of nerve inflammation and when you awaken in the morning with a stiff neck. Heat a little St. Johnswort oil (five to ten tablespoonsful) in a small pot, but never let it boil! Soak a piece of cotton in the oil and apply it to the painful spot. *Note: check carefully that the oil is not too hot; however, it should be as hot as the patient can take it.* Then cover it with a small piece of toweling and secure it with a bandage or scarf. If the area is on the neck and shoulders, put on a tightly fitting undershirt.

Internal Use of St. Johnswort Oil

St. Johnswort oil can even be employed internally to good effect for an upset stomach and for gastrointestinal catarrh. Persistent constipation can even be treated by taking St. Johnswort oil, since it lubricates hardened intestinal contents. It has also been found that St. Johnswort oil heals and relieves pain when the gastric and duodenal mucosa are irritated as a reaction to stress. The only problem in this respect is that St. Johnswort oil has a rather individual odor and flavor, and when several teaspoonsful are taken, it can cause uncomfortable belching to occur for a long time. Therefore we recommend that for internal treatment the oil be taken in capsule form; the capsules dissolve in the small intestine and spare you the taste and discomfort.

St. Johnswort oil even proved an important aid during the birth of our three children (see page 211).

In his medical writings, the great physician, alchemist, and medical reformer Paracelsus sang a hymn of praise for St. Johnswort in which he described its antidepressive effects and various methods of preparation and applications. We find his enthusiasm entirely contagious!

> There is no herb in the German nation, nor in any other lands, that can be held in higher esteem in the preparation for the healing of

wounds than this herb. And its virtue cannot be described; how great it is and how great are its uses. And in all formulas there is no medicament that is so good and without detriment, without hazard, as the healer St. Johnswort. And it is not possible that a better medicament could be found for the wounds in all the lands. And all books for healing wounds are nothing compared to St. Johnswort, for its virtue shames all formulas and doctors, they may cry as they may. . . .

❧ 10 ☙

HEALING HERBS
FOR HEADACHES

*The Earth is a very patient teacher. One of Her most
important teachings is to be patient.*
> Wabun, companion of the
> Chippewa healer Sun Bear

The single most important thing to understand about headache is that
it is not a disease. It is a symptom. As natural healers, we do not wish
to suppress symptoms, but rather endeavor to get at the root cause. We
urgently implore you not to "combat" a headache with painkillers.
Perhaps a little story will make the point.

What Is a Symptom?

Let's assume that you have a freezer at home. One day, a warning light
flashes, telling you that something is wrong with the appliance. You call
your local repairman; he comes, looks at the freezer, and begins to work
on it. Finally, he opens the housing surrounding the little red warning
light and removes the bulb. He then tells you that he's repaired the freezer:
"See, the little red light doesn't shine any more." Would you settle for
such a "repair"? Surely not. But exactly the same thing happens when
you take a painkiller drug for a headache, a laxative for chronic constipation, or sleeping pills for insomnia. All you are doing is taking out the

little red warning light, the signal that's telling you that something deeper is amiss.

Pain is an alarm signal. It is a cry from your body for attention. If you do not provide that help but instead rebuff every new pain with a chemical drug to "kill the pain," you will eventually create a state of permanent pain. In the United States alone, several million people are afflicted with chronic headache.

HEADACHE HAS VARIOUS CAUSES

If you suffer from headaches only occasionally or rarely, they are usually associated with some other disorder. For instance, an *upset stomach* with nausea and vomiting can announce itself with a bad headache. The solution is simply to treat the underlying complaint, and the headache will disappear: drink peppermint tea or some other stomach tea, Swedish Bitters, or balm tincture (see also chapters 9 and 12), and/or apply a Swedish Bitters compress to the upper abdomen (see pages 105–107).

Incidentally, it goes against the grain of natural healing to suppress the urge to "throw up." Quite the contrary: this natural method of expulsion was followed by physicians in earlier times with good success, since the process triggers a wide range of compensatory mechanisms in the solar plexus and the gastric system. Most adults have a horror of vomiting, whereas children seem more ready to accept relief through it. Our experience has shown that in many cases of stomach trouble, nervous stomach colic (often caused by great excitement or fear), and migraine, the condition is appreciably eased immediately after vomiting takes place.

A *gastric infection* can also be the cause of headaches. Here, help can be obtained from mallow tea, sage tea, and linseed and Swedish Bitters compresses (see pages 105–107 and 167–169).

It is well known that *high blood pressure* can also be a source of headache as well as of tinnitus (ringing or buzzing in the ear). Here the symptoms gradually disappear if the blood pressure is reduced by means of a long-term mistletoe cure and an adjustment of the patient's diet (see page 144).

In cases of *chills and severe head colds,* the general feeling of debility is often accompanied by headache and chronic inflammation of the sinuses and parasinuses, resulting in severe pressure pains in the head that can last for days. Immediate relief is obtained by rubbing eucalyptus oil or oil of peppermint onto the forehead and temples and by inhaling these with the nose directly at the neck of the bottle or in the form of a hot vapor bath. All the measures described in chapters 6 and 7 concerning the immune system and colds are to be recommended for this type of headache: echinacea drops, thyme baths, chamomile vapor inhalations, and Swedish Bitters compresses on the forehead.

Chronic constipation must also be mentioned along with the nutritional causes of headaches. Here relief is naturally to be found in bulk- and fiber-rich whole foods. You cannot attempt to achieve regularity by continually taking drastic chemical—or even herbal—laxatives! Such treatment is sure to produce severe side effects (see also pages 175–176). People who suffer sluggish bowels, and thus dull headaches as a result of incorrect diet, almost always take too little exercise. This results in a sluggishness of the whole metabolism, overweight, and loss of energy and performance—in short, a vicious circle that must be broken in some way. We propose that headaches should be viewed as alarm enough to encourage us to change our habits and lifestyle.

In view of the continual increase in *allergic disorders* nowadays, it is not surprising to discover that headaches are often precipitated by allergens (substances that trigger allergic reactions). Such headaches are usually accompanied by other symptoms—swelling of the mucosa, respiratory distress, dermal eruptions, and so on—and do not require a separate or specific treatment other than the removal of the allergen. However, if headaches appear as the only sign of an allergic reaction to particular substances in the food or air, years often pass by before the connection is revealed. In any event, an attempt should be made to cleanse and desensitize the body to allergens by fasting and by blood-cleansing cures (with Swedish Bitters, stinging nettle, and blood-purifying teas; see chapter 5).

It seems almost unnecessary to mention the fact that *chemical medications* often cause headaches as a side effect and can be the cause of allergic reactions. Ironically enough, severe headaches can even be caused by headache tablets. This is a case of actual intoxication. Uwe Henrik Peters and Kurt Pollak, the authors of an excellent book entitled *Vom Kopfschmerz kann man sich befreien* (*You Can Free Yourself From Headaches;* Munich, 1976), have reported seeing patients in their headache clinic who became trapped in the vicious headache circle because their consumption of painkillers had led to habituation and tablet ad-diction. The only possible relief here is the complete withdrawal of pain-killers plus careful naturopathic treatment, including the use of natural nerve tonics and psychotherapy.

In some cases, the *eyes* are the cause of headaches. If your vision is poor or if your spectacles or contact lenses are no longer effective, overstrain of the eye muscles can be the cause of headaches. Obviously, the solution is to correct these problems. If you still experience periods of feeling tense or eyestrain, we advise you to make a Swedish Bitters eye compress (see page 104). This is also a perfect treatment for eye ir-ritation due to new contact lenses.

For women who frequently suffer from *premenstrual headaches,* a tea of cowslip flowers has proved particularly useful. (See also pages 204–206.) The tea should be drunk not only when the symptoms ap-pear, but three times daily for a period of several months. If during meno-pause headaches occur frequently and in combination with other typi-cal symptoms, we recommend a tea blend of equal parts: St. Johnswort, balm, hops, and passion flower (see also page 210).

We are certain that the majority of headaches are due to stress. However, what one person experiences as stressful, another can con-sider great fun! It is important to understand that each individual per-son will have his or her own conditions or "definition" for stress. In any event, stress can be reduced by measures that generally strengthen and calm the nervous system. Particularly relaxing herbal baths prepared with balm, valerian, and lavender bring the "equalization" and balance we desire (see also page 113). In the previous chapter we listed several tea blends designed to build a stable nervous system from which it is pos-sible to master and even enjoy most of life's tensions (see pages 114 and 115). Here is another formula that can be used when you feel exhausted or find it difficult to concentrate. Instead of becoming self-critical or force-fully "pushing" yourself, simply take a break and prepare the following tea. Enjoy one to two cups and then return to what you were doing.

❧ Vitality Tea ❧

4 parts masterwort root
3 parts damiana leaves
3 parts hawthorn leaves with blossoms
3 parts rose hips

3 parts rosemary leaves
3 parts hibiscus flowers
1 part maté
1 part ginger root
½ part ginseng root

This aromatic tea will liven you up and really help you to cope with a variety of stressful situations. It's perfect for replacing coffee and common tea when you want a little stimulation in the morning or throughout the day without damaging your nerves.

MIGRAINE

Severe chronic headache and the typical migraine attack are classic examples of psychosomatic disorders, which can be ameliorated and improved by physical therapy and the use of herbs but cannot be healed in the real sense of the word so long as the underlying emotional problem is unknown and unresolved.

The "Migraine Type"

Dr. Uwe Henrik Peters, director of the Neuro-Psychiatrische Universitätsklinik in Mainz, West Germany, has characterized the patient of the "migraine type" as a person who is very precise and conscientious, loves order, and feels an above-average sense of responsibility at work. The migraine type has a strong need for security and feels threatened by the unknown, and thus tries to avoid uncertainty as much as possible. Interestingly enough, attacks of migraine are very often precipitated by situations of nervous expectation before social events.

The migraine type is not an ideal leader but rather makes an indispensable right hand. For such people, the problem is how to relax and release the day's tensions. It is not accidental that many migraine attacks occur on the weekends, in the evening, and at the start of vacation periods. As soon as such a person begins to relax, deep and hidden anxieties rise up from the subconscious and then are immediately repressed. The "migraine type" is a rational thinker. He or she cannot accept the irrational, especially when expressed as his or her own doubts, fears and worries, and so on. These anxieties and the need to repress them eventually result in severe attacks of pain.

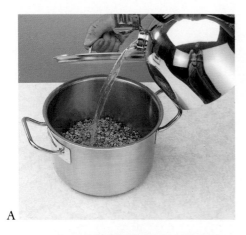

A

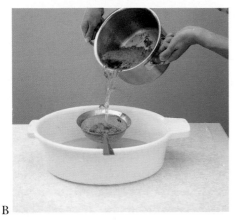

B

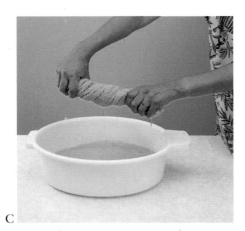

C

FIGURE 10

Chamomile Back Compress

A. Pour boiling water over chamomile flowers and allow to steep.

B. Strain off the herbs and pour the infusion into a shallow container.

C. Soak a small terry cloth towel in the infusion (holding it by the ends to avoid burning fingers) and wring out carefully.

D. Place the towel over the patient's back, shoulders, and neck (as hot as can be tolerated).

E. Soak a second small terry cloth towel in the infusion, wring it out, and place it on top of the first towel.

F. Turn both towels over so that the fresh one covers the skin. Take off the upper towel, soak it in the infusion, and repeat steps E–F.

G. Massage reddened skin with St. Johnswort oil and have the patient rest or take a nap.

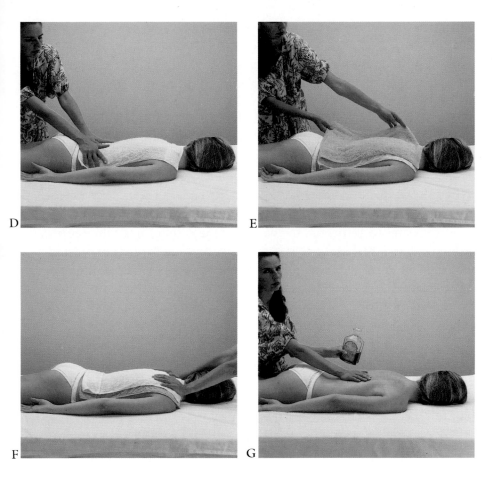

D

E

F

G

Migraine Symptoms

The body processes that take place during a migraine attack consist of vasoconstriction in the brain, often accompanied by heightened sensitivity to light, flashes before the eyes, nausea, a desire to vomit, and severe muscle spasms of the back and neck. These myospasms usually make an appreciable contribution to the occurrence of the attack; yet if they are systematically treated it is very possible to reduce the frequency of the attacks independent of the psychological trigger mechanisms.

Chamomile Back Compresses for Migraine

Hot chamomile compresses really work wonders for the relaxation of painful, tense muscle nodes and fibers. Prepare a strong infusion with a full cup of chamomile flowers and two quarts of water, cover with a lid and allow to steep for about ten minutes, then strain off through a sieve (see figure 10). In the meantime, get the patient to lie on his or her stomach and gather together the following equipment: a large, wide pot with the prepared herbal infusion, two small terry cloth towels, and a bottle of St. Johnswort oil. Dip one of the cloths into the infusion, wring it out, and place it spread out as hot as the patient can tolerate it on the back, shoulders, and neck. Then soak the other towel in the hot infusion, wring it out, and place it on top of the first towel. Now turn both towels over so that the fresh, hot compress is against the patient's skin. Remove the upper towel and soak it in the mixture. Repeat the procedure (soaking the towels and so forth) ten to twenty or more times until the patient responds with a real sense of relaxation and a genuine loss of tension, evidenced by deepened breathing and many deep sighs. The skin will be very reddened by this process and should be massaged with St. Johnswort oil afterward. Rest or a nap should follow the treatment. It is utterly unbelievable how relaxing and comforting this treatment can be. The same procedure yields excellent results even if only hot water is used, and it is also an effective preparation of the muscles for other, subsequent treatments, such as massage or chiropractic manipulation. However, the cramp-reducing effect is increased when the chamomile infusion is used.

It should be noted here that few migraine patients are willing or able to make the time and effort to undergo such a compress treatment as a preventative measure. If, however, a partner, relative, or friend can persuade him or her to do so, the compress procedure will be supplemented by the additional healing effect of physical touch and loving care from another person. We have observed dramatic results from this element alone. For further discussion of this subject, see the book *Touch For Health,* by John F. Thie (Marina del Rey, California, 1973).

In cases where the migraine patient has no help from another person, a treatment with a red-light (infrared) heat lamp is another possibility for removing tension from the back and neck. This is easy to arrange and is also very comforting.

Migraine Tea
We have had wonderful results in migraine patients from the following tea blend:

Migraine Tea

6 parts rosemary leaves
4 parts peppermint leaves
4 parts balm leaves
4 parts sweet violet
3 parts feverfew
½ part sweet violet flowers

This tea has a very fine flavor and so can be enjoyed daily for many months. It is also recommended as a morning wake-up drink or breakfast tea, since the essential oil of rosemary causes vasodilation, promotes peripheral blood flow, and generally stimulates and refreshes. It was Paavo Airola, the author of *How To Get Well* (Phoenix, 1974), who wrote that violet leaves and flowers are effective against migraine. Homeopathic teachings and Paracelsus—and the tradition of herbology with him—agree that sweet violet, which hides from the sun and loves the shade, can be of help to migraine patients who cannot tolerate bright sunlight and seek darkness and shade.

FEVERFEW

Feverfew (*Chrysanthemum partenium*) is a medicinal plant used in headache therapy that has caused a great stir since its rediscovery in England. A few decades back there were reports of migraine sufferers who reduced their attacks by chewing one or two leaves of the plant on a daily basis. But two new double-blind studies carried out in London support the theory that taking the leaves of feverfew prophylactically can reduce or prevent migraine attacks. Today, it is used as a simple tea or in tea blends.

ROSEMARY

Rosemary (*Rosmarinus officinalis*) is a typical Mediterranean herb that has been employed medicinally in those warm countries for thousands of years. The evergreen rosemary bush has gnarled, woody twigs and branches, needle-shaped leaves, and delicate, pale blue flowers. In countries with cold, snowy winters it can be cultivated in the garden but must be well protected from the harshness of winter. It is the fragrant leaves and young shoots that are employed medicinally. They contain, above all, essential oil and a camphorlike substance that stimulates the blood flow.

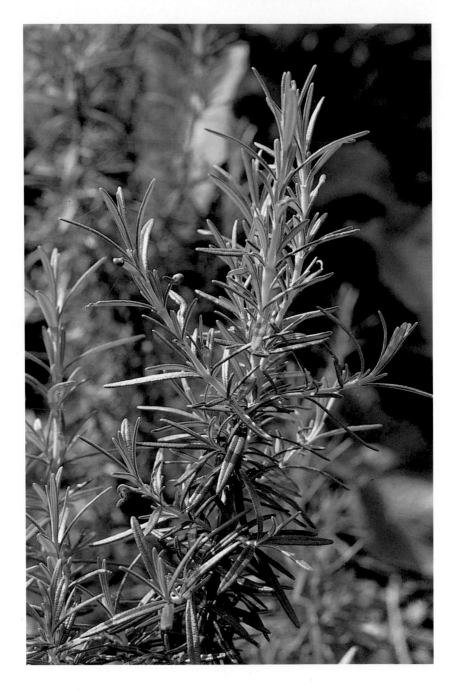

ROSEMARY   *Rosmarinus officinalis*

Tradition holds that rosemary "warms the body from the inside out." This tonic effect is exploited in bath preparations made from rosemary leaves or oil of rosemary. A rosemary bath is refreshing and stimulating when you are mentally and physically fatigued and can be highly recommended as a preventative measure for persons liable to headaches. When added to a shower gel or soap, rosemary enlivens you and makes you more active. This herb is effective when taken internally as a tea or extracted in rosemary wine and when used externally in baths or washings. It promotes blood circulation, tones up the vessels, invigorates, warms, and increases your awareness.

Rosemary wine helps sufferers from low blood pressure, elderly people who lack exercise, the convalescent, and all who are suffering from fatigue and a general lack of dynamism (for the recipe, see pages 148–149). Furthermore, the external application of *rosemary extract* for supportive treatment of muscle and joint rheumatism has been scientifically confirmed. Taken internally, rosemary helps against a bloated feeling, flatulence, and mild spasmlike disturbances of the stomach, intestines, and gall bladder. *Expectant mothers, however, should not drink rosemary tea,* but certainly they can enjoy a warm, refreshing rosemary bath. Rosemary is also popular as an aromatic and flavorful culinary condiment.

TEAS AND BATHS FOR HEADACHE

Since people who tend toward headache build up too much internal tension, we recommend not only Migraine Tea but also various other teas, tinctures, and baths that have a nerve-calming and -strengthening effect. Teas containing equal parts of valerian, balm, and hops; or tea of St. Johnswort; and baths with balm, lavender, or valerian can promote relaxation and "switching off" before the point of overtension (and hence the start of a migraine attack) is reached. Smoking would naturally be catastrophic for such patients, for nicotine is known not only to damage the nerves but also to constrict the blood vessels.

INSTEAD OF A PAINKILLER

Before you choose to take a headache pill or painkiller, try a natural method to alleviate discomfort. Take a walk in the fresh air; rub peppermint oil, or eucalyptus oil, a camphor-containing ointment, or arnica tincture on the forehead and temples (see also page 217). You can also apply a cool Swedish Bitters compress on the forehead and neck, or a water application such as a cool- or cold-water face effusion.

Another natural "aspirin alternative" is the rosemary foot-bath. The temperature should be increased slowly by adding hot water. After about ten minutes, the feet are taken out of the hot water and plunged directly into cold water (waiting in a bucket or deep pan right next to the hot rosemary bath). With this treatment tension and frozen energy will be drawn down to the feet, away from the head, and, as simple as this may sound, will bring great relief in many cases of headaches. All the other external applications mentioned work by cooling down the head area directly, yet this method seems to bring the best results. Do not judge this before you try it yourself!

Fasting Therapy

Severe, repeated attacks of headache or migraine can quite often cease in amazing fashion through fasting, carrying out an intense blood-cleansing cure, or changing to a whole-grain, fresh-food diet containing no animal protein. (See also pages 42–43.) Headaches are very often a sign of a blockage in the metabolic system, which can be overcome by the tedious removal of poisons and wastes along with proper intake of vitamins, minerals, enzymes, chlorophyll, etc.

Dietary Therapy

"Adjustment of the diet" is certainly one of the most difficult therapeutic measures to carry out. Departing from habitual eating patterns and tastes built up over a lifetime not only requires self-observation and analysis but demands resolution, determination, willpower, an understanding of biological relationships, and more. In addition to all that, you will have to be prepared to deal with the intense feelings and emotions of "withdrawal reactions," similar to those faced by the new non-smoker. This may amount to a whole new way of being!

We are often asked what kind of diet we recommend. We propose a lacto-vegetarian whole foods diet with lots of grains (both cooked and raw), whole grain breads, lots of vegetables and raw salads, excellent quality vegetable oils, fruits, nuts and seeds, plus dairy products and eggs.

This is how we prepare our family meals at home: everything is fresh and homemade with no industrially refined or prepared foods. With our children we take great care to reduce foods and drinks containing sugar to a minimum. However, if we are invited to someone's home or if we are going out for dinner, we enjoy eating fish or good meat as well as a fine glass of wine or champagne. It seems to us that the quality is what matters most. This is why we buy our foods from organic producers or health food stores. We also find that such a diet must be masterfully cooked and must taste delicious and be presented attractively; otherwise it simply becomes too boring. We always like to experiment and especially enjoy incorporating elements of nouvelle cuisine into our meals.

Having tried out various strict diets ourselves, we think it is most important not to overdo any diet philosophy. This is especially true for children, who usually cannot take extremes well and when they are old enough tend to rebel against any restrictive dietary regimen. A wider and more varied diet of natural foods can be delicious and fun to prepare, and is certainly preferable to having the children sneak off to spend their allowances on forbidden treats and junk foods. When choosing your ideal diet, it is also important to consider the culture, climate, seasonal changes, and of course your own unique lifestyle and constitution.

Please remember that a headache is always an indication of something deeper within yourself being out of balance. By all means, use natural treatments to relieve the pain and discomfort, but do not forget to reveal and treat the real cause of the problem.

∾ 11 ∾

HEALING HERBS FOR
HEART AND CIRCULATION

*If you are not ready to alter your way of life, you
cannot be helped.*

Hippocrates

The topic of heart complaints, arteriosclerosis, and cardiac infarction
is one of the most explosive issues of our day. At the turn of the
century, 4 percent of all deaths in Germany were caused by diseases of
the heart and circulation. Today, these problems account for more
than 50 percent of the death rate, and cardiac infarction is the most
common cause of death. In 1987, 986,000 people died of diseases of
the heart in the United States—twice as many as the number who suc-
cumbed to cancer, and 55 percent of all deaths due to degenerative
diseases. Because of the real and present danger involved in acute cardiac crisis, this entire field must be reserved for the medical doctor.
*Self-medication is advisable only in the case of complaints where the
doctor has excluded the possibility of an organic disorder.* However,
medicinal herbs deserve all the more regard in this connection as means
for preventing the occurrence of conditions that encourage cardiac
infarction, mainly slowly developing arteriosclerotic changes of the
vascular system.

For all that, it still must be said that the "big guns" of heart treat-

138

ment are fired far too often, probably as a result of the habitudes of doctors today, as well as the hard sell and hype of the pharmaceutical industry. In 1984 the German magazine *Stern* carried a story about the "slow poisoning of the nation," in which it reported that three million West Germans regularly took digitalis preparations without really needing to. The cost of this—about 116 million dollars—is borne by Germany's public health insurance program. The worst part of the story is that ninety thousand of those hooked on digitalis are suffering from intoxication; ten thousand, moreover, have had to be hospitalized in order to treat disease symptoms resulting from the digitalis medication itself.

HERB FOR THE HEART: HAWTHORN

In any event, herbal medicine can provide an excellent, proved medication for the treatment of mild cases of cardiomuscular weakness and cardiac rhythm disturbance by way of hawthorn (*Crataegus oxyacantha* and *Crataegus monogyna*). The delicate white blossoms and small leaves of the hawthorn tree or bush can be used as a heart-strengthening tea. Its red, ripe berries are used as well, rarely for tea, but rather as a tincture in numerous proprietary preparations. We find hawthorn either cultivated or "gone to the wild" around gardens and in field hedgerows. In autumn it is a favorite with birds, who love to eat its berries.

An herbal monograph on *Crataegus* published by the Deutsches Gesundheitsministerium (German Federal Health Authority) confirms the experience of traditional medicine: hawthorn invigorates the heart when its performance is diminished and lessens the feeling of oppression in the heart region. It is particularly suitable for elderly people whose coronary vessels are subject to sclerotic constriction and whose heart muscles are no longer optimally supplied with blood. Anxiety, palpitations, tightness in the chest, gasping for breath, and the rapid onset of fatigue during physical effort are all signs of this condition. Elevated blood pressure is another accompanying symptom.

Two or three cups of hawthorn tea (made from the leaves and blossoms) taken daily give the older heart the support it requires and reduces blood pressure as well. This is the reason why hawthorn is included in many geriatric tonics (preparations to increase the physical and mental capacities of older people). Hawthorn should be taken on a long-term basis to yield the best results, for numerous clinical investigations and studies have revealed that symptoms were appreciably improved after about six weeks of treatment. Fortunately, hawthorn tea or tincture can be consumed for months or even years without producing any negative side effects. Hawthorn is often employed in homeopathic preparations as well, both by itself and in combination with other substances. The fields of application here are also for cardiac weakness, the "aging heart," cardiac rhythm disturbances, angina pectoris, circulation problems, and blood pressure disturbances.

Hawthorn is also employed with great success to invigorate the heart after other kinds of damage have occurred, such as following surgery and during convalescence while recovering from severe infectious diseases. We can also recommend that people who have suffered a heart attack take hawthorn tea and tincture. In such cases, hawthorn supports convalescence and is effective for the prevention of further infarcts as well. Hawthorn should still be taken even when the prescription of a cardiac glycoside is unavoidable, since according to Max Wichtl, professor of pharmaceutical biology at the University of Marburg, it has been observed empirically that the dosage of cardiac glycosides can be reduced when they are combined with hawthorn tea or drops. Thus, if the potential side effects of powerful cardiac medications can be reduced by lowering the dosage, the opportunity should be grasped by everyone involved.

Hawthorn can also help younger people avoid damage when their daily life is very hectic and subject to extreme stress. The typical executive of about forty, who holds down a stressful job, takes too little exercise, and perhaps smokes and does not eat a balanced diet, is in very great danger of sooner or later suffering a cardiac infarction and should definitely drink one or two cups of hawthorn tea every day as a precautionary measure. Please let us note, however, that herbal medicine should never serve as a preventive merely to enable someone to continue an unhealthy lifestyle. In this context, we hold with the remark made by Hippocrates that serves as an epigraph to this chapter.

An excellent heart tea blend in which hawthorn is augmented by motherwort and nerve-soothing herbs such as balm and St. Johnswort is particularly recommended for men and women who are continually subject to stress.

❧ Heart Tea ❧

8 parts hawthorn leaves and blossoms
4 parts St. Johnswort
4 parts balm leaves
2 parts motherwort
2 parts mistletoe

The "nervous heart" also responds quite well to the above mixture; by this we mean people who react to weather changes, excitement, and overexertion with nervous heart symptoms, unease, and palpitations. For the nervous heart, we also highly recommend the following "heart drop" prescription developed by our pharmacist colleague Mannfried Pahlow. It is compounded from four very effective herbal tinctures:

❧ Heart Drops ❧

4 parts spirit of balm (Spiritus Melissae Comp.)
2 parts valerian tincture (Tinctura Valerianae)
2 parts peppermint tincture (Tinctura Menthae Piperitae)
2 parts hawthorn tincture (Tinctura Crataegi)

In the case of acute nervous heart complaints, take twenty to thirty drops in a little water; relief can be experienced quite quickly.

OTHER NATURAL TREATMENTS

A counterirritant treatment with cold water is also most helpful in cases of nervous heart. Lay a wet washcloth on the chest over the region of the heart as a cool heart compress, or dip the feet in cold water for three minutes and dry them with vigorous rubbing. You can also immerse the arms in a washbasin filled with cold water for about three minutes. These cold-water treatments are all refreshing and clear both the head and heart. *They should not, however, be employed by people with high blood pressure.*

HIGH BLOOD PRESSURE

High blood pressure (hypertension), which affects elderly people in particular, is another disorder that has almost become "epidemic" in industrial countries as a result of an unnatural lifestyle. Here, it seems

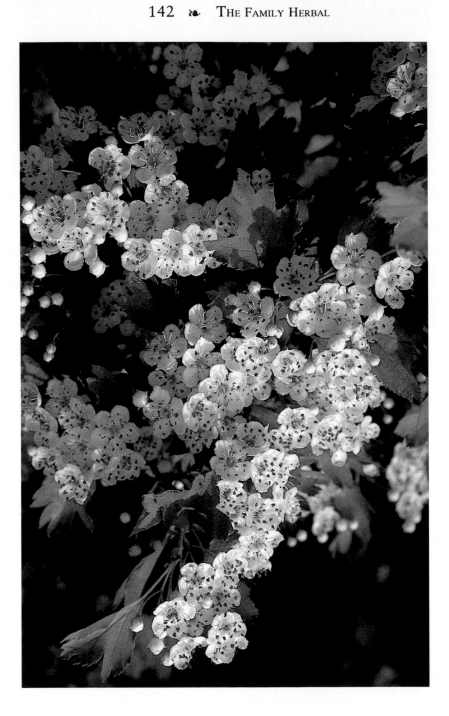

HAWTHORN   *Crataegus monogyna*

clear that many years of incorrect diet is the major causative factor. Hence, adjustment of eating habits to a low-salt, whole-food natural diet with plenty of fresh, raw foodstuffs and grains can achieve a great deal.

Patients whose blood pressure is too high are generally mesmerized by their blood pressure readings and tend to overlook the fact that hypertension is not in itself a disease but a symptom—in addition to which it is a marvelous equalization mechanism of the body.

Here, the body is striving to keep the material transfer between capillaries and tissues at the levels necessary to maintain the nutrition and function of every single cell with all the means at its disposal. If the cell walls of the capillaries have become less permeable because of arteriosclerosis, and if the blood has thickened, then the body naturally increases the blood pressure. This is a vital and very sensible reaction. Preventing or diminishing this action by reducing the blood pressure symptomatically with antihypertensives is, therefore, a quite dangerous artificial intervention in the body's purposeful, life-maintaining regulatory processes. Moreover, the side effects of chemical antihypertensives range from dizziness and confusion to severe liver damage, hematological changes, recurring headaches, and cramps.

Hawthorn's closest companion is garlic, and both substances are recognized as nontoxic and mild healing agents for the treatment and prevention of hypertension. In the case of hawthorn, scientists ascribe the antihypertensive effects to the choline and acetylcholine it contains. The fact that fresh garlic can prevent arteriosclerotic changes and blood thickening has recently come under much public discussion and has been borne out by clinical testing. Garlic's wild relative, ramsons, works in the same manner, and both the cultivated and the wild species are medicaments that can be highly recommended to elderly people. (See also page 53.) A sufficiently high dose level is decisive for success. People with heart and circulation problems would have to eat one or two cloves of fresh garlic each day; therefore, many use one of the more convenient, commercially available preparations instead.

Two herbs that are also used to treat high blood pressure, but about which science and folk medicine are in disagreement, are mistletoe and shepherd's purse.

Mistletoe

Mistletoe (*Viscum album*) is a very idiosyncratic plant surrounded by age-old traditions of ancient cults and magic rites. It is an evergreen semiparasite that grows primarily on deciduous trees. Its seeds are eaten by birds, digested, excreted, and thus transferred to other trees without ever touching the ground. Today we still find traces of Celtic mistletoe worship in the traditional rites surrounding the mistletoe bough at Christmastide in England and many other countries. According to herbal tradition, mistletoe tea is able to reduce elevated blood pressure and remove such symptoms as dizziness and the sensation of blood rushing to the head.

Since 1907 many pharmacological and clinical studies of mistletoe have been conducted, but as yet science has not found an adequate or acceptable explanation of the effectiveness of mistletoe tea. In fact, according to Dr. Wolfgang Holzner of the College of Agriculture, Vienna, analysis of the plant reveals the presence of substances with antihypertensive effects (viscotoxin and acetylcholine), but thus far the scientific viewpoint has been that these substances would be effective only if injected intravenously, because the result of oral administration would either be nonabsorption or destruction in the gastrointestinal tract. According to Dr. Hans Becker, professor of pharmaceutical biology at the University of Saarbrücken, studies of mistletoe's action have yielded evidence that "the action occurs via an effect on the autonomic nervous system."

Shepherd's Purse

Findings are similar in the case of the herb known as shepherd's purse (*Capsella bursa-pastoris*). Pharmacological investigations have also revealed here that the active ingredients are organic nitrogen compounds (choline, acetylcholine, tyramine), which as a result of their effects on the nervous system reduce blood pressure even when present only in tiny quantities. According to current scientific opinion such substances can be effective only when they are injected, but not when they enter the gastrointestinal tract through the vehicle of tea. Nevertheless, traditional folk medicine attributes to shepherd's purse the ability to act in a regulatory and equilibrating manner on both the aging heart and the blood pressure, whether it is too high or too low. In addition, this unprepossessing plant is said to be an excellent agent for stanching bleeding of all kinds. (For more information, see pages 200–201, 203.)

In our pharmaceutical practice we have had good results reducing blood pressure with mistletoe tea and with a blend of hawthorn, shepherd's purse, and mistletoe, both for reducing elevated blood pressure and for raising it when it gets too low.

❧ Blood Pressure-Regulating Tea ❧

8 parts hawthorn leaves and flowers
6 parts mistletoe
6 parts shepherd's purse

Please note that Mistletoe Tea and Blood Pressure-Regulating Tea are not prepared like regular herbal teas, because mistletoe herb is hard and tough, like a root. Add four teaspoonsful of herb to two cups of cold water, allow it to soak overnight (about eight to ten hours), heat up to drinking temperature (warm, not hot or boiling, because some of mistletoe's active ingredients would then be destroyed), and consume only in the morning on an empty stomach. Two cups per day is the correct dosage. In contrast to common opinion, mistletoe herb (deprived of its berries) is completely nontoxic. However, much higher doses may cause gastric irritation.

For the sake of completeness, it should also be mentioned that mistletoe is sometimes employed for the treatment of cancer, mainly in anthroposophic medicine (a branch of homeopathy based on the teachings of Rudolf Steiner). Various complicated extracts of mistletoe, which are employed exclusively by doctors in the form of injections, have proved an effective means to combat pain, especially during postoperative treatment, and to inhibit the growth and spread of cancerous tumors. It also appears that such mistletoe preparations affect the immune system by activating the lymphocytes. Injected mistletoe extracts are also employed successfully to treat degenerative inflammatory joint diseases such as rheumatism and arthritis.

LOW BLOOD PRESSURE

As we have already mentioned, low blood pressure can also be regulated by the very same herbs that affect high blood pressure: mistletoe and shepherd's purse. This is a phenomenon that an artificial, chemical

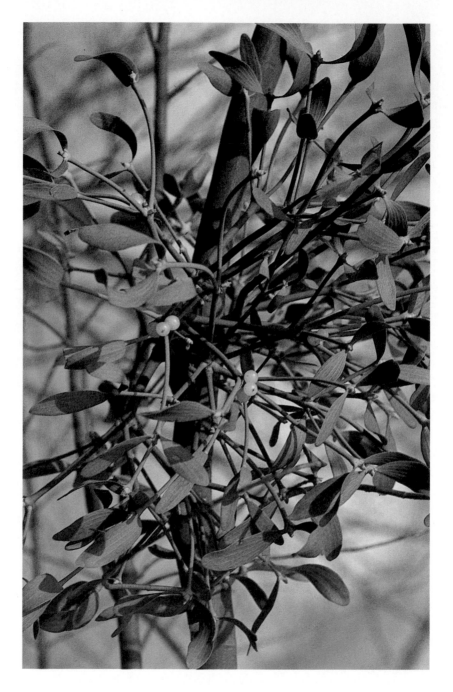

MISTLETOE · *Viscum album*

drug could never imitate. By design, its effect would be too limited to a particular reaction mechanism to be able to guide the body back to a natural state as herbs can. If hypotension (low blood pressure) causes problems, two cups of coffee or common tea in the morning can be a help as well. The less frequently these beverages are employed, of course, the stronger their effect will be. Our opinion is that coffee and "black tea" should not be used on a daily basis, but as a medication only when the situation merits. They can be good mild stimulants for low blood pressure. Regular physical training over long periods, open-air sports, (e.g., jogging), and movement therapy cause the unpleasant symptoms associated with low blood pressure to disappear in the most natural manner possible. In any case, statistics show that people with low blood pressure live longer than people with normal or raised blood pressure.

However, when it comes to heavy conditions of tiredness and exhaution due to coronary and circulatory weakness, as can often be observed after long diseases, operations, or during menopause, we recommend a tincture of hawthorn berries and camphor. Furthermore, this medication works wonders in situations when menstrual cramps, extremely low blood pressure, heart palpitations, or irregular pulse lead to circulatory collapse and fainting. The immediate intake of ten drops restores heartbeat and pulse to normal rates within a very short time and so helps the patient to speedily overcome the crisis (or prevent it). Patients with a chronic tendency to become faint (more often women and teenage girls) take ten drops three times a day on a regular basis.

❧ Drops Against Fainting ❧

19½ parts tincture of hawthorn berries
½ part camphor

INSUFFICIENT BLOOD CIRCULATION

Peripheral circulatory problems are often experienced by the elderly or people who engage in little physical exercise in the feet and lower legs as well as the hands and arms. This shows as a numbness, prickling sensation, and lack of energy, often resulting in an inability to move these limbs. For this entire area of complaints we recommend rosemary and lavender. They are both able to tone up the whole body, vitalizing not only the blood circulation but the entire nervous system by virtue of their strong essential oils. Rosemary and lavender fragrance all by itself has a clearly stimulating, awakening, and refreshing effect. With lavender and rosemary you can make pleasant teas, but even more effective may be their external use in the form of invigorating full baths, foot or arm baths, or washings.

Rosemary and lavender are also ideal in cases of either physical or mental exhaustion and when blood pressure irregularities need to be balanced. For an invigorating full bath, place 1½ cups of rosemary and ½ cup of lavender in two quarts of water and bring up to the boiling point. Cover and allow to extract for ten to fifteen minutes; then strain and add the extraction to the bath water. For a partial bath, simply use smaller amounts of herbs and water. Convalescent patients and apathetic, sickly children feel wonderfully stimulated by a rosemary-lavender bath; their facial color improves, and they suddenly become more active and alive.

Father Sebastian Kneipp, the great German natural healer, praised rosemary above all herbs and valued it as a warming, stimulating, and heart-strengthening herb. (For a full description of rosemary, see pages 133–135.) In the case of peripheral circulation problems, alongside the various methods that promote vigorous local circulation, such as saunas, alternating hot and cold footbaths, showering with hot and cold water, brushing down, breathing exercises, and gymnastics, a good deal of help is brought about by rubbing the affected limbs with rosemary tincture, particularly if the patient is confined to bed or otherwise unable to move (see also page 135).

In our pharmacy, we also prepare rosemary wine. It is a pleasant-tasting favorite, especially among our older customers. A small glass every morning and evening has a strengthening effect on the blood vessels and acts as a general tonic. (With respect to the efficacy of herbs extracted in wine, please see pages 39–40.) Here is the recipe:

~. Rosemary Wine .~

10 parts rosemary leaves
4 parts hawthorn berries
2 parts hawthorn leaves and blossoms
½ part raisins
½ part ginger
½ part St. Benedict thistle
½ part cinnamon bark

½ *part St. Johnswort*
½ *part yarrow flowers*
½ *part comfrey root*
½ *part melilot*
½ *part oats*
½ *part horsetail*

Mix all the ingredients in a big glass container or widemouthed bottle, then add a little over two quarts (two liter bottles) good white wine. Let the extraction take place over a period of ten days; shake well every day, then strain the liquid and store in a tightly sealed dark glass bottle. Rosemary wine is a delight not to be missed! If you ever have the occasion to visit elderly friends who are just recovering from a difficult health problem, this is the tonic to bring! They'll love it and use it, and it will give them a little pep and add a bit of color to their cheeks.

LAVENDER

Lavender (*Lavandula angustifolia*), like rosemary, is one of the ancient herbs that traveled across the Alps from Mediterranean regions. The outstanding fragrance of its tiny flowers has made it a favorite addition to soaps, cosmetics, and body care products as well as perfumes. In the days of ancient Greece and Rome, distinguished ladies of society used extracts of lavender in their toiletries.

Today, lavender is a very common, much-loved garden plant. Its thin silvery leaves form thick shrubs, above which the taller stalks with violet flowers grow. Lavender is a rich-blooming summer plant that is best harvested in July and August. It is easy to grow in sunny places and is cultivated in huge fields, especially in southern France. If you have it in your garden you should collect and dry some of the flowers to use them in baths, tea mixtures, herbal pillows (see pages 115–117), or potpourris, those delicate-smelling niceties of English gardening culture. In our grandmother's time, little sachets of lavender flowers were still much in use for disinfecting cupboards, chests, and drawers, and for keeping away moths and other insects from clothing and bed linen.

Lavender is also an effective medicinal herb. Its strong and refreshing odor derives from its very high content of essential oil. Lavender flowers have a calming effect on the central nervous system, which is why they are often used as an ingredient in nerve-calming teas. As a

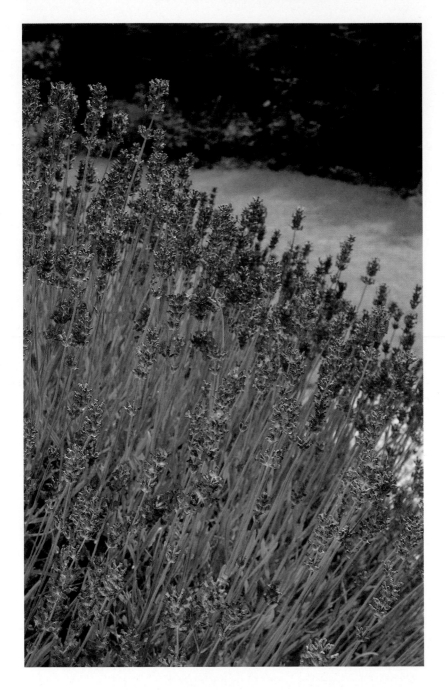

LAVENDER   *Lavandula angustifolia*

therapy for autonomic nervous disorders, they are most often used as a bath rather than a tea.

Lavender flowers not only help you relax and calm down but also invigorate, refresh, stimulate, and vitalize. People with low blood pressure should try a lavender full bath every other evening to get rid of such unwanted symptoms as buzzing in the ears. Women with low blood pressure who become pregnant (in which condition the blood pressure tends to go even lower) will find lavender baths to be very helpful and perfectly safe as long as they do not bathe in water that is too hot. For patients who are confined to bed for long periods of time, it can make a world of difference to be bathed once a day with a lavender-water sponge bath. This pleasant and natural stimulus can be made as a decoction of one handful of lavender flowers in a quart of water, or can be prepared by simply adding a few drops of lavender oil to the bath water.

~ 12 ~

HEALING HERBS
FOR DIGESTION

*Let your foods be your medicines and your medi-
cines be your foods.*

Paracelsus

Our digestive system is an absolute miracle of precision and coopera-
tion, a system that astonishes anyone who studies it intensively. Even a
few simple facts about our digestive system read like the entries from a
book of world records. Our stomach produces approximately one to
two quarts (liters)of stomach acid per day. The food we eat travels a
distance a little over 26 feet (8 meters) within our bodies. The small intestine, the place where our food is actually decomposed and resorbed,
is 19 to 21 feet (6 to 6½ meters) long. Its total surface area is greater
than that of a tennis court, for the inner walls of the small intestines are
covered with millions of tiny, finger-shaped villi. Together these minute
projections increase the surface area of the small intestines to more than
360 square yards (300 square meters). The cells that make up the villi
are rapidly consumed, and therefore millions and millions of these cells
must be replenished daily.

In the mouth cavity alone there are 100 trillion microorganisms.
The entire digestive tract is populated by truly symbiotic bacteria whose
job it is to break down the "nutritional broth" and decompose it by

fermentation. The important role of these beneficial bacteria was only made evident in the early twentieth century when medicine began to employ massive amounts of antibiotics and sulfonamides that radically exterminated them. The absence of a healthy physiological bacteria population in the intestines creates a favorable environment for candida, a yeast disease widely distributed in industrialized countries and most extremely in the United States. This disease—one that has grave consequences for the whole human organism—is an excessive penetration of a weakened and depleted intestinal flora by yeasts (*Candida albicans*) and is the exclusive result of humankind's misuse of chemical medications for more than fifty years. It can be reliably healed by a careful "new cultivation" of physiological bacteria.

Although we do not have sufficient experience in treating conditions of candida with herbal medications, as this disease has only come to our attention since we became involved with the health care problems of the United States, we do have some indications that the classic "digestive" herbs—fennel, caraway, and anise, as well as bitter roots such as angelica, sweet flag, and centaury tops—would be appropriate to support such a cure. The main part of this therapy must certainly be a proper diet (no sugar at all!) including a well-dosed intake of acidophilus preparations. However, the above-mentioned herbs, used as teas, can help to prepare the right "milieu" within the intestines so that the physiological bacteria are able to thrive and the pathological ones are discouraged. For the present, we are watching these therapies closely so that in the near future we will be able to give our own best recommendations for persons suffering from candida.

Besides the immediate effect of malnutrition and various symptoms of indigestion as the consequence of a depleted intestinal flora, it is well known these days that the intestines, with their physiological bacteria population, play a key role in our immune system. It is no exageration to call the intestines the main immunological organ. This means that resistance to infections depends directly upon a person's health and the good condition of his or her intestinal tract.

CAUSES OF DIGESTIVE PROBLEMS

The three main triggers for digestive problems and disorders of the intestinal tract are a faulty diet, stress, and strong medications. In fact, many allopathic physicians regard this as the field par excellence for phytotherapy, simply because chemical pharmaceuticals are often ruled out as therapeutic agents because of their potentially damaging side effects, particularly those involving the liver, stomach, and intestines.

Logically enough, the digestive tract—along with the teeth and gums—is the first system of organs to suffer from the effects of faulty nutrition. Thus a broad long-term therapy of the digestive organs requires a change in eating and drinking habits. Such a change is mandated, not merely because of an unhealthy or wrongly composed diet (too much protein, sugar, white flour, and preserved and refined foods and not enough grains, raw greens, vegetables, etc.), but also because of a faulty attitude toward food and eating. Not taking the time to cook or eat properly; "grabbing a bite" while busily working, reading, or watching television during meals; not being able to relax when eating; irregular eating patterns; eating while tense or feeling stress; not chewing well; compulsion about calorie counting (particularly among women)—these are the kinds of bad habits that can often trigger disorders.

FOUR GROUPS OF DISORDERS

The manifold and interlocking symptoms and disorders of the digestive system can be divided roughly into the four following groups.

First we may list the diffuse stomach disorder, stomachache, and pain spasms in the region of the stomach and small intestines, and colic of the stomach, intestines, and gallbladder. All the above may occur as a single episode or in the form of recurring complaints. These disturbances are the result of irritation, inflammation, or ulcer formation, whereby the organs concerned exhibit hyperactivity and great irritability; in other words, they have excess energy.

The second group is made up of loss of appetite, a bloated feeling, flatulence, and inability to tolerate certain foods. These are disorders based in digestive weakness where too little digestive juices are produced, where the digestive organs are not active enough; that is, they have too little energy.

Third, there is the "upset" stomach, which is often the result of infection, accompanied by nausea and a desire to vomit. When such infections occur in the intestines rather than in the stomach, the result is often intestinal colic with acute or chronic diarrhea. These disorders occur particularly frequently as a result of outside influences such as consumption of tainted food or the effect of travel to distant countries (with resultant dramatic change in climate, environmental conditions, and diet).

The fourth and certainly the most common of all digestive disturbances is constipation, which in its chronic form affects 10 percent of the population or more. Women are afflicted by it more often than men.

THE HEALING FAST

When discussing disorders of the digestive tract we feel we must point out once again the beneficial aspects of a healing fast. Total abstinence from food for one or more weeks means that since the digestive organs have almost nothing to accomplish, they have the chance to rest and regenerate completely. Conditions of energy deficit as well as those involving too much energy react very positively to a period of fasting. We also know from our cultural and religious history that holy and spiritually-motivated persons have regularly employed periods of fasting for meditation and inner preparation for an upcoming mission or quest. It must be emphasized here again that a healing fast is not merely abstinence from food. Various measures for cleansing and purification and a careful buildup of the diet afterward are also required in order to create true health. (See also pages 41–43.)

POSITIVE ASPECTS OF VOMITING AND DIARRHEA

Spontaneous emptying of the digestive tract in the form of diarrhea or vomiting can be very beneficial in the sense of self-healing our bodies. If we have eaten rancid fat or tainted fish, for instance, and our stomach rids itself of this poison by vigorous vomiting, we should be thankful. Similarly, when the small or large intestines react to toxins in the nutritional broth with watery diarrhea, this can, under certain circumstances, be a lifesaving reaction. For this reason the natural healers of earlier generations such as Christopher Hufeland and Bernhard Aschner, as well as the physicians of the ancient world, used to employ purgatives in the initial treatment of many disorders (such as feverish colds) and thus deliberately brought about vomiting or diarrhea in order to stimulate the body to conduct a thorough process of excretion. These practitioners held it to be one of the greatest errors of the medical arts to miss the correct moment for the administration of the purgative. Even today, though such methods seem a bit strange to us, we should at least acknowledge that our body does react sensibly when it rejects the unacceptable in this manner, and we should not overreact by "stopping" the diarrhea or suppressing vomiting. In cases where you have the feeling that you have eaten something that does not agree with you (such as tainted shellfish, rancid oil, or spoiled meats), the only correct thing to do—and the most natural as well—may be to encourage vomiting.

We have already mentioned that children react much more naturally and directly in this connection and usually recover quickly after spontaneous excretion (see page 126). On no account should you force a person suffering from digestive disorders to eat when he or she does not have the appetite. Anxious mothers often make mistakes here because of the worrisome loss of weight of a small child. In such circumstances with our own children we always made certain that they drank plenty of herbal tea, but we did not feed them until they insisted on wanting something to eat; and from that moment on they always exhibited a healthy appetite and were perfectly fine in less than a day.

Care is really required only with small children (one to three years old) and particularly with babies (up to one year old). *Infants with acute diarrhea must have prompt medical attention.* In cases of prolonged vomiting or diarrhea the body loses too much water and salt, and it is necessary to combat the danger of internal dehydration. Older children may be treated with continual supplies of peppermint, chamomile, or fennel tea with a pinch of salt (because salt binds liquid to the body). If your two- or three-year-old children refuse the salted tea, we are able to recommend the following trick we learned from our homeopath: allow them to eat as many salty pretzel sticks as they want. (Do you know any child who doesn't love pretzels?)

CHILDREN'S STOMACHACHES

When a child in our family complains of stomachache and voluntarily lies down, our first step is to give him or her a cup of peppermint tea and a Swedish Bitters poultice on the abdomen. If it is the beginning of an inflammation or a digestive disorder caused by consuming unfamiliar food or overeating, then sipping the warm tea and the comfort created by the blood flow-increasing poultice generally eases the pain and everything is usually back to normal the next day. This recommendation naturally applies to adults as well (see pages 105–107).

FIRST GROUP OF DISORDERS: IRRITATION AND INFLAMMATION

Heartburn and gastritis (inflammation of the gastric mucosa), both of which are caused by excess stomach acid, are almost always chronically recurring disorders. Even when they occasionally disappear for weeks, months, or even years, in 80 percent of the cases they reappear in conditions of particular stress. Such conditions express themselves as gnawing, burning, or coliclike pain in the upper abdomen. People with such disorders should drink three to five cups of the following tea (Stomach Tea No. 1) daily. It is best to space out the drinking of this tea over the whole day. It is also wise for these people to drink the tea even at times when no unwanted symptoms are present.

🍃 Stomach Tea No. 1 🍃

8 parts angelica root
4 parts chamomile flowers
4 parts balm leaves
4 parts peppermint leaves
2 parts caraway seed
2 parts fennel seed
1 part wormwood

Because it contains balm leaves, this blend is also effective against disorders of nervous origin. When it is evident that the pain is a result of emotional problems, such as overexcitement, worry, anger, or mourning, we recommend that in addition to the tea either St. Johnswort oil (one teaspoon mixed in milk or soy milk, three times daily), or St. Johnswort oil capsules (five capsules, three times daily) be taken. (See also page 123.) In cases of severe gastritis or gastric ulcers, whereby the patient not only suffers severe pain, but also has a feeling of total exhaustion, simple chamomile tea is a wonderful help. Also a mixture of chamomile and calendula flowers or chamomile flowers and balm leaves, drunk lukewarm and unsweetened, reduces pain quickly.

We can say from our own experience that when we suffer from such abdominal pains and have neither appetite nor pleasure in eating, we fast for a short period of a half or a whole day and continuously drink tea from just these three last-named herbs. After such a period of special care, the stomach and intestines are completely calmed.

The following tea mixture has a very good effect as well. It also has a most pleasant flavor and thus has the advantage that it can be offered to the entire family (perhaps with the evening meal) as well as to the stomach patient.

❧ Stomach Tea No. 2 ❧

4 parts yarrow
4 parts peppermint leaves
4 parts St. Johnswort
4 parts balm leaves

It should be self-evident that people with sensitive stomachs should abstain from coffee, tea, nicotine, alcohol, and all ice-cold beverages. It is our experience that to avoid these substances—especially the last named—is almost impossible in the United States! Most stomach patients will have had their own experiences with these substances and will be willing to give them up of their own accord. But it is not quite so self-evident that they should also avoid sugar (in the form of baked goods, chocolate, candies, sweetened drinks such as soda pop and cola, etc.). You should know that aside from its other health-damaging effects, white sugar lures acid from the stomach, hence patients suffering from excess acid should avoid it at all costs (see also pages 93–94). Fresh or dried fruits or pure unsweetened fruit preserves are a marvelous replacement to satisfy almost any sweet tooth.

Stomach Ulcer

The stomach ulcer is considered to be a very typical executive complaint. Yet it can also be triggered in housewives, children, and even babies by continual exposure to mental tension and stress. Not only hunger but also anxiety and anger cause the vagus nerve to transmit impulses to the stomach that stimulate the secretion of gastric juices. This connection was clearly observed in Europe during World War II, when unusually high numbers of soldiers suffered from stomach ulcers. Today, the feeling of always having to do five things at once or of being continually under time pressure colors the daily life of almost every stomach patient.

In contrast to the pains that characterize other digestive disorders, those of stomach ulcer are usually marked by the fact that they often disappear immediately after eating but then get worse thirty minutes to two hours following the meal. *Anyone who has symptoms of this type should go for a medical examination to rule out the possibility of stomach cancer.* If this is the case it is sensible to solve the problem with both relaxation methods and medicinal herbs. Although herbs can help, however, obviously they cannot remove the emotional stress or fear that is causing the problem.

Chamomile Roll Cure

A very successful method of treatment for stomach ulcer—one that is fully recognized by academic medicine in Germany—is the so-called roll cure with chamomile tea. For this a strong infusion is prepared from three teaspoonsful of chamomile flowers in a cup of water. This tea is drunk warm in the morning on an empty stomach. Then the patient lies in bed on his or her back for ten minutes, then for ten minutes on the right side, next on the left side for ten minutes and last directly on the stomach for ten minutes. Finally, a warm stomach compress made with chamomile tea is laid on the stomach, and the patient rests on the bed for at least half an hour. This entire procedure is repeated every day for ten days. Throughout the day, Stomach Tea 1 or 2 as the sole beverage taken should be drunk in sips. The roll cure can also be made with equal parts of chamomile flowers and balm leaves.

Chamomile Compress

To make a chamomile compress, prepare an infusion from a handful of chamomile flowers in one quart of boiling water. Cover with a lid and let steep for ten minutes. When the infusion is cool enough to touch, take a large piece of cotton (big enough to cover the stomach area) and soak it in the infusion. Squeeze out the excess liquid and place the moist compress directly on the skin of the stomach. Cover it with a large towel and wrap a woolen scarf or piece of flannel around the area. The abdomen of the patient must be kept warm, so the procedure is best done in bed. Do not allow the compress to lower the patient's temperature by leaving it insufficiently covered.

Linseed and Mallow Infusions

Mucilage-containing herbs such as linseed and mallow act in a somewhat different manner on the same disorders. When they are properly prepared, the mucilage released gently coats the inflamed mucosa and protects it, safeguarding it from irritation by gastric acid and nutrient broth.

Please note that linseed for the treatment of gastritis, enteritis, and colitis (inflammation of the mucosa of the stomach or the small or large intestine) is prepared differently and has a different effect than when it is employed for the treatment of constipation. (For comparison, see page 177.) In the cases discussed here, four to six teaspoonful of linseed must be crushed for mucilage preparation and covered with a cup of hot water or milk in a small bowl. A mucilaginous mass is formed within ten to twenty minutes; this must be drunk or eaten with a spoon (depending on the amount of liquid used) at least three times daily one half hour before meals.

When mallow is employed, the tea must be prepared as a cold infusion: pour a cup of lukewarm water over two heaping teaspoonful of herb. Allow to steep for five to ten hours (or overnight), warm the infusion slightly, drain off, and drink warm. (Do not on any account use boiling water; otherwise the valuable mucilage will be destroyed. For more information on mallow, see pages 89–91.)

A Story About the Use of Linseed

I myself (Barbara) experienced an absolutely convincing demonstration of the healing powers of linseed when I was a young girl and spent six weeks in Tunisia with a group of French and Tunisian student friends. We were all guests of Tunisian families, and without a thought I ate the exotic food, which was extremely spicy for European tastes, and drank local water the whole time. After about four weeks my digestion had just about given up the ghost—that is, everything I ate passed straight through my system just as it went in. As a result of the unaccustomed spices and bacteria, my intestines had totally lost their ability to digest and assimilate food. After my body began to feel somewhat shaky and occasionally grew feverish, I began to be concerned about my state of health. Following the well-meant suggestions of others to eat only white rice did not bring any improvement.

When the holidays came to an end, I returned home rich in experi-

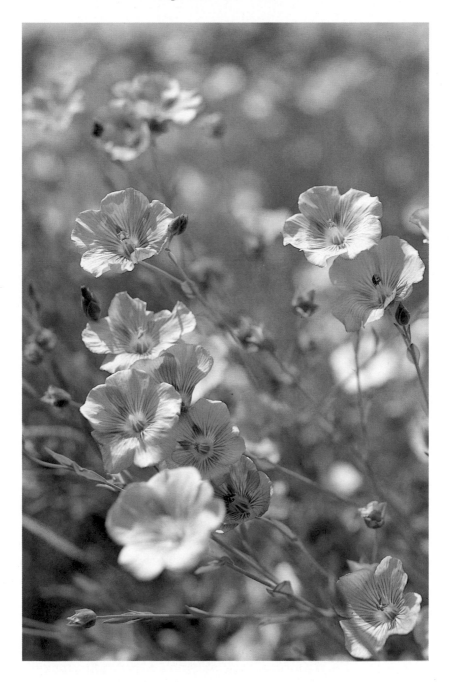

FLAX   *Linum usitatissimum*

ence and unforgettable memories, but still unable to retain any food in my system. I then adopted a diet consisting of a porridge of crushed linseed in warm milk with a teaspoonful of honey several times a day: it was the only food my intestines would accept. When the watery diarrhea subsided after a few days, I began to consume plenty of yogurt along with the linseed porridge and recovered totally within a week. It was only years later that I realized how dangerous the situation had been for me then and how miraculously the linseed had helped me.

The Flax Plant

Flax (*Linum usitatissimum*) is a very imposing cultivated plant that humanity has known for thousands of years (see page 161). Linseed, the seed of the flax plant, has a delicate, clear light blue blossom on a long, slender but very tough stem bearing many narrow delicate leaves along its length. Findings of linseed in excavations of ancient lake dwellings have shown that even our prehistoric ancestors used flax seeds as a food. Flax was also cultivated in fields by the ancient Egyptians, and the fibers of its stem were creatively processed into the finest linen cloth. The ancient Greeks preferred linen robes, and it is known that Roman legionaries were proud of their linen chest "armor," which provided excellent protection from minor injuries. The severe competition presented by the cheaper cotton displaced the cultivation of flax throughout almost all of central Europe toward the end of the nineteenth century. However, linen and flax are now enjoying a renaissance. The botanical name of this plant means "the most useful flax" (*lin* is the Old English word for "flax"). Flax seed is not only a superior food (with an extremely high content of desirable unsaturated fatty acids) and healing agent, it is also the source of linseed oil, which is today as in former times the base for many paints and lacquers. Real linoleum (who would have thought it?) is also manufactured from linseed oil.

SECOND GROUP OF DISORDERS: INDIGESTION

Now let us turn from the digestive disorders that are characterized by excess of energy in the form of hyperirritation, hyperacidity, inflammation, and hyper-motor activity to those in which there is a lack of activity and energy, where the tissues are cold and sluggish and react slowly. Here the front-line medications are the bitter herbs. We have already discussed their effects in chapter 8 (pages 93–95) in connection with Swedish Bitters elixir. They are an important group of medicinal herbs known to pharmacists under the collective name "Amara." These substances are further subdivided according to the accompanying substances that modify the bitter flavor into either pure bitters, mucilage-containing bitters, or aromatic bitters (these last are the ones that also contain essential oils). Such herbs help in cases of generally poor digestion and sluggish stomach with insufficient acid production. They also generally arouse the appetite and stimulate the production of gastric juices. In the following tea mixture, centaury and angelica (for more on the latter plant, see pages 97–99) are the protagonists, mixed with other herbs to harmonize their flavor and effect. The tea blend has a pleasant taste in spite of the bitter herbs.

🗫 Digestion Tea 🗫

4 parts peppermint leaves
3 parts angelica roots
2 parts caraway seeds
2 parts chamomile flowers
2 parts balm leaves
2 parts St. Johnswort
2 parts cloves
2 parts centaury tops
1 part cassia bark
½ part lavender flowers

Centaury

If you saw the small and lovely light pink flowers of centaury (*Centaurium erythraea*) growing in a sparse pasture or on the grassy edge of a forest you would never believe that this pretty little flower could taste so extremely bitter. But since it belongs to the gentian family (the medicinal plant *Gentiana pannonica* is the most bitter herb we know of), it is among the most highly valued herbs known to pharmacists as "Amara pura." Centaury is harvested as *herba,* whereby the bitter substances are most concentrated in the flowers. This is the reason why in English the dried herb is referred to as "centaury tops." We counsel you *not to collect centaury yourself,* because at least *in Europe, it has become a very rare plant in danger of extinction.*

CENTAURY   *Centaurium erythraea*

Centaury supports weak intestines and a slackened, "tired" stomach that does not produce enough stomach acid. *Please note that a stomach with overacidity would not benefit from centaury.* The symptoms could possibly worsen in the latter case; hence it is important first to discover exactly what the malfunction of the stomach really is. An acid stomach usually is accompanied by repeated sour belching and frequent heartburn, whereas the weak stomach hurts only when it is filled and does not have sufficient energy to function properly and provide the required amount of acid secretion. Centaury clearly stimulates the appetite, and has been observed by our colleague Mannfried Pahlow to be effective even in the condition of anorexia nervosa, the psychogenic aversion to eating food that is seen almost exclusively in women and adolescent girls.

In keeping with the general properties of bitter herbs, centaury also stimulates the autonomic nervous system and thus the function of the heart and general blood circulation, and therefore helps in conditions of nervous exhaustion. For gallstone patients it is an effective medicinal that calms irritated gallbladder and prevents colic. Those who do not mind its bitterness can use centaury tea, which is best prepared as a cold infusion and warmed slightly before drinking.

Insufficient Bile Production

Very often a digestive weakness shows itself as an inability to digest fatty foods. Some people have a clear aversion to fats, and some get feelings of pressure in the stomach area or experience heavy flatulence after eating foods rich in fats. If this is the case, you should drink Liver and Bile Tea before meals regularly to stimulate the production and excretion of bile.

Bitter herbs such as St. Benedict thistle seeds, wormwood, and dandelion roots stimulate the secretion of all digestive juices including saliva, gastric juices, and pancreatic juices. Our Liver and Bile Tea is principally made up of bitter herbs, but it is palatable because of the other herbs that are blended together with them.

❧ Liver and Bile Tea ❧

7 parts dandelion root with herb
3 parts St. Benedict thistle seeds
3 parts raspberry leaves
2 parts centaury tops

(continued on next page)

2 parts yarrow flowers
1 part cat's foot flowers
1 part angelica root
1 part boldo leaves

In the case of disorders of the liver, gall bladder, and pancreas, dandelion root and herb alone in the form of tea, tincture, salad, or as freshly pressed juice is also to be highly recommended (see pages 46–48).

All bitter herbs are recommended not merely for long-term treatment of chronic gastrointestinal weakness, but also as a general tonic and regenerative for convalescent patients recovering from infections, for the elderly, and for those whose autonomic nervous system is weakened by exhaustion and unable to react properly. People of weak general constitution (so-called asthenic types) usually react very positively to a long-term treatment with bitters. For example, bitters brings about stimulation of cardiac activity and increases the circulation of the blood with improvement of the blood flow to the internal organs, particularly the mucosa of the stomach and the intestines. *Nevertheless, even these natural healing agents should not be overdosed,* otherwise habituation will lead to their having the opposite effect. No more, but also no less than three to four cups of Liver and Bile Tea or Digestion Tea prepared in the normal way should be drunk daily. Here it is important to allow the bitters to act on an empty stomach; hence the tea should be taken first thing in the morning and before meals. Swedish Bitters Elixir is ideal for people who require strong digestive stimulation. In such cases, a teaspoonful of elixir should be added to each cup of tea (see pages 101–103).

Peppermint

Peppermint (*Mentha piperita,* also *Mentha aquatica* and *M. spicata*) occupies a special position among the herbs that act on the stomach, intestines, and gallbladder. Its active principle is the essential oil, which in its isolated form is employed against colds and chills as well. Although peppermint is scarcely bitter in flavor, it is nevertheless an Amarum aromaticum and is characterized by its powerful bile-stimulating effect and by its ability to stimulate stomach and intestinal functions, both of which are typical of bitter substances. For this reason, peppermint is the herb of choice for children and difficult patients who refuse to take bitter teas or elixirs, because it has an extremely fine flavor and is refreshing and stimulating as well. It is also a perfect stomachic when nausea and the urge to vomit are present. For the treatment of stomach ulcers, however, its effectiveness is the subject of much controversy.

Warm peppermint tea drunk in sips brings rapid relief from cramplike pains of the stomach and intestines, particularly when they are accompanied by flatulence and foul-smelling, foamy stools. The same is true when diarrhea is present along with the cramps. Last, but not least, a tea made from peppermint leaves promotes the production and of flow of bile, calms the irritable gallbladder, and lessens the pain of an acute gallbladder attack. Peppermint leaves also provide an excellent taste corrective whenever there is the need to improve the taste of a tea mixture. It adds a touch of freshness to every herb combination (see the recipes on pages 241, 243, and 249).

True peppermint is a hybrid, as are many other valuable mint species. They can be readily cultivated in your garden, which we recommend highly, because this enables you to conjure up many attractive and refreshing delicacies with fresh mint leaves (see pages 250–251).

Gallstones

Here are a few hints for sufferers from gallstones. Patients with this condition have told us time and again how well bitter-tasting teas work for them. Here you must simply accept the bitterness; attempts to sweeten such a tea only make it more unpleasant. The following blend is a tea that relaxes cramps and can help avoid gallbladder attacks.

❧ Gallstone Tea ❧

6 parts peppermint leaves
4 parts centaury tops
4 parts balm leaves
4 parts fumitory
2 parts wormwood

Linseed Compress for Gallstone Colic

We have also had good experience with the pain-ameliorating effect of linseed compresses in addition to peppermint tea in cases of acute gallbladder attack. For this purpose, put crushed linseed (about 7 ounces, or 200 grams) in a small cotton bag (in emergencies a folded pillowcase

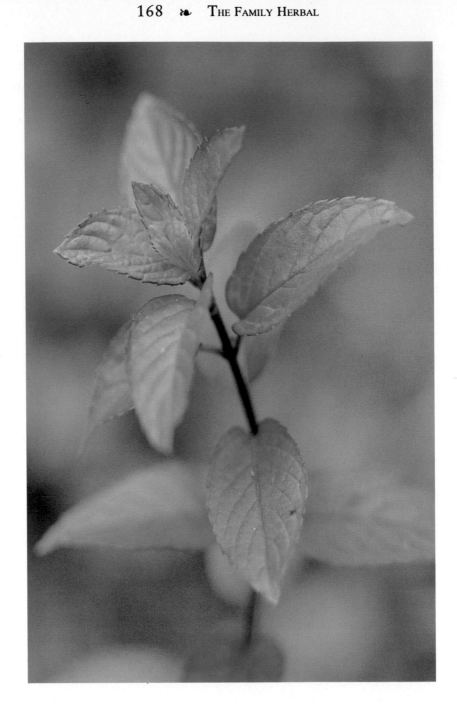

PEPPERMINT   *Mentha piperita*

will do) and hang it in a tightly closed pot of boiling water for about ten minutes. Allow the bag to cool slightly after removing it from the water and apply it directly on the patient's skin (as hot as he or she can bear it) where there is the greatest pain. Then wrap the abdomen with a woolen scarf or cloth to secure the bag. The compress should be allowed to act for about thirty minutes. Its comforting warmth, which penetrates into the depths of the body, has often made painful colic subside in the most astonishing way. These linseed compresses can also provide excellent supportive therapy for liver inflammations and swollen liver. Moreover, they are wonderful for babies and small children who are querulous and restless because of stomachache. (See also the recommended treatment for children's stomachaches, pages 156–157 and 172–173.)

For inflammations of the gallbladder and bile duct we recommend the following basic tea:

Tea for Gallbladder Inflammation

4 parts centaury tops
4 parts peppermint leaves
4 parts yarrow
4 parts chamomile flowers

This basic formula may be varied depending on the nature of the symptoms. If flatulence is present, then add fennel and caraway; if a feeling of pressure regularly occurs at meals (an indication of a blockage of bile flow or too little bile production), add yellow gentian and dandelion root; if there is simultaneous constipation, add a small amount of buckthorn bark and a few senna pods.

Prevention of Gallstones

People whose gallstones occasionally trouble them or who have already undergone surgery for this condition naturally seek means of preventing the further formation of gallstones. The versatile dandelion has proved itself here once again. It has been established scientifically that dandelion combats the formation of new stones and the growth of existing ones as well, even though it has not yet been completely explained how this can happen. Hence our recommendation in chapter 5 (page 48) to undertake a cure with fresh dandelion leaves, or dandelion tea made from root and herb, applies particularly to sufferers from gallstones. Such a cure, if it is to be effective, means drinking three cups of tea daily over a period of six to eight weeks twice a year; one of the cups of tea can be replaced, if desired, by dandelion salad. (Incidentally, when it is prepared with imagination and variety, dandelion salad is a true gourmet's delight.)

Flatulence

The problem of flatulence and feeling bloated after eating points either to a general weakness of the digestive organs and glands or to the fact that the various digestive juices are not ideally adjusted to each other. Here too, very specific herbs are indicated, which are mainly employed in blends with other digestive herbs. These are—along with the bitter herbs—caraway (*Carum carvi*), fennel (*Foeniculum vulgare*), and anise seed (*Pimpinella anisum*). In each case the healing power is concentrated in the essential oil. Caraway grows both cultivated and wild, while fennel and anise are only found in cultivation. However, they look quite similar, so that advanced botanical knowledge is required to tell the three apart or to distinguish them from other wild flowers such as wild carrot. These three seeds are much loved as spices—and not without reason, for they are able to make breads, cakes, potato recipes, and vegetable dishes much more easily digestible and appealing. If flatulence alone is to be treated, then a tea should be prepared from the seeds of the three herbs as follows.

❧ Flatulence Tea ❧

8 parts caraway seeds
6 parts fennel seeds
6 parts anise seeds

It is very important to open the seeds by crushing them briefly with a mortar and pestle or milling them for a few seconds in a food processor, blender, or coffee mill, so that the essential oils can be extracted into the water. Allow the mixture to steep for about ten minutes, and don't forget to cover the extraction in order to contain the volatile oils. Without the crushing of the seeds it would require hours of steeping to bring about the proper extraction (see also pages 211–212). If other digestive herbs or roots are to be included, it will be worthwhile to break the three types of seeds open separately and then brew them together with the other

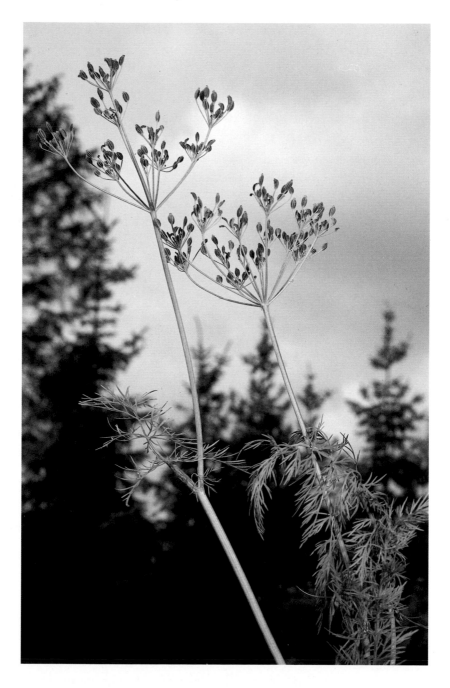

CARAWAY *Carum carvi*

herbs, or else prepare the entire mixture as a cold infusion, letting the roots and seeds soak overnight. The following blend makes a flatulence tea that is very mild and pleasant tasting and has proved its value many times over, especially for infants and children.

❧ Wind-Releasing Tea for Babies and Children ❧

5 parts fennel seed
5 parts caraway seed
5 parts chamomile flowers
5 parts peppermint leaves

When adults have a bloated feeling and suffer from flatulence they can use the following, somewhat stronger tea.

❧ Wind-Releasing Tea for Adults ❧

4 parts fennel seed
4 parts caraway seed
4 parts yarrow
4 parts angelica root
2 parts anise seed
2 parts centaury tops

It should be unnecessary to point out in connection with these symptoms the necessity for a proper diet of fresh, nutritious whole foods. Unfortunately, it is true that a damaged, lax digestive system that has become accustomed over decades to refined and overcooked food will react at first to whole grains and raw food with definite unacceptance and severe flatulence. Most people in this state tend to reject whole food after a first attempt, instead of trying patiently to retrain their stomachs, intestines, and digestive glands. Since the digestion of whole food requires more effort, these organs must be slowly restored to a state of enhanced vitality and natural activity.

Treating Flatulence in Babies and Small Children

Flatulence connected with stomachache is often a serious problem in very young infants and occasionally in babies up to one year old; their continual crying and inability to fall asleep often brings young, inexperienced mothers and fathers to the brink of despair. For the sake of these parents, we will summarize the methods that we found to be successful with our own first baby (our two daughters never had symptoms of this sort) as well as with countless children we have encountered in our practice.

1. *Wind-releasing tea for babies and children* (see page 172). Give it to the baby unsweetened by the teaspoonful or in a bottle as often as he or she wants it.

2. *Linseed compress* (see pages 167–169). If your baby has severe stomachache this method is most effective in combination with the above-mentioned tea.

3. If the linseed compress seems too difficult or cannot be made for other reasons, *a simple compress with hot water or chamomile infusion* (see page 159) on the baby's abdomen will also help. As with all hot compresses, you must work fast enough so that the child will not get cold. You can also use a heating pad or hot water bottle instead, but the linseed compress and chamomile compress are both superior.

4. In the case of very small babies who habitually cry before falling asleep, it often helps to *lay a sachet containing dry chamomile flowers on the abdomen*. The sachet must be big enough to cover the child's entire stomach area. The essential oil being released from the flowers gives comfort and relaxes cramps and soon lets the baby sleep peacefully.

5. In the case of children over nine months, and particularly those between one and five years old, *a warm bath with yarrow* is an especially effective treatment in cases of stomachache and flatulence. While in the bathtub, the child can also drink chamomile, peppermint, or yarrow tea or the Wind-Releasing Tea for Children.

THIRD DISORDER: DIARRHEA

Now let us turn to acute diarrhea. When diarrhea is accompanied by pain or colic, relief can be brought about by various teas such as chamomile tea or linseed porridge and (in the same way as for children) by applications of warmth to the abdomen (hot water bottles, heating pads, moist hot compresses). When it is truly necessary to "stop" diarrhea (see page 156), we recommend either grated apple or dried blueberries. Dried blueberries, long used in Europe for this purpose, are scientifically recommended as a medicament in nonspecific acute diarrheal disorders. The determining factor in successful treatment is the amount that is taken; take three to seven teaspoonful daily and

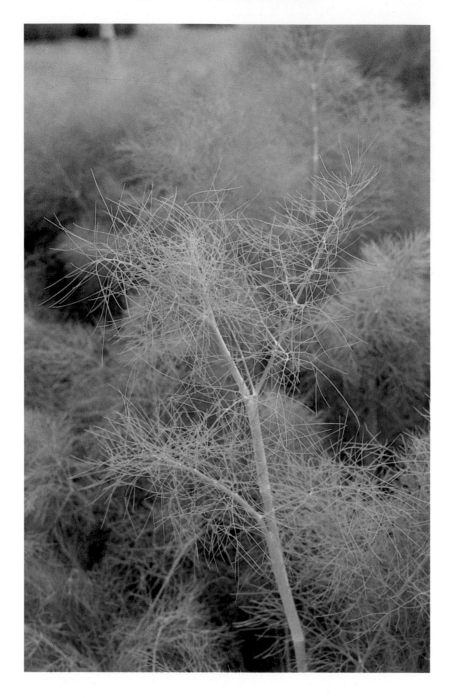

FENNEL   *Foeniculum vulgare*

chew them very well. The same applies to grated apples (but please use only organically cultivated ones); the diarrhetic patient should eat a total of about two pounds over the course of a day. Grated apple alone (along with plenty of herbal tea) makes an excellent diet that will quickly enable the patient to recover. Once the diarrhea has ceased, it is advisable to fast for a day and then gradually build up the diet again starting with apples, carrots, and rice.

FOURTH DISORDER: CONSTIPATION

The last section of this chapter is devoted to the topic of constipation. The widespread incidence of chronic sluggish bowels and constipation is an alarming disease of modern civilization, one that is almost entirely attributable to too little exercise and the usual poor diet. The putrefying bacteria usually present in the intestines as a result of bowel sluggishness means that the entire organism is continually flooded with toxins, which promote the occurrence of various states of severe, chronic disease.

The Dangers of Laxative Herbs

It is true that among the medicinal herbs are several that have a more or less drastic effect in that they stimulate intestinal peristalsis. *All herbs of this type contain so-called anthraquinones and have damaging side effects* (just as mineral laxatives do) if they are taken regularly for a prolonged period of time. *Their chronic use can lead to habituation and/or counterregulation,* so that the laxative becomes ever less effective, higher and higher doses are required, and the bowels stray further and further away from the ideal state of self-regulation.

Studies have revealed that the chronic abuse of laxatives, including herbal ones, leads to disturbances of the electrolyte equilibrium and can result among other things in potassium deficiency. This condition in turn opens the way for possible weakening of the heart muscles and of the skeletal musculature as a whole. A vicious circle is created here in that potassium deficiency also weakens the intestinal muscles and these lose ever more tone. In Germany, the law requires that the labels on all anthraquinone preparations must bear a warning that possible potassium deficiency can intensify the effect of chemical heart drugs (cardiac glycosides). In the future a caution will also have to be included stating that such laxatives should not be taken during pregnancy or while breast feeding. We also want to mention that many of the more drastic laxatives irritate the intestinal mucosa, so that heavy doses can cause chronic inflammation.

For all these reasons, we provide a recipe for a laxative tea only with the proviso that because of the above factors *it is to be used only to treat occasional constipation, and must not be used for the treatment of chronically sluggish bowels.*

❧ Laxative Tea ☙

5 parts senna pods
5 parts buckthorn bark
4 parts senna leaves
2 parts raspberry leaves
2 parts fennel
1 part peppermint leaves
1 part calendula flowers

Chronic habitual sluggishness of the bowels can be treated with absolute effectiveness and no risk by the consumption of sufficient fiber and ballast materials, even when it has been present for many years. Milled whole-grain porridge is a very simple recipe that will cure every constipation within three days; it has been recommended for decades by such renowned European dieticians and naturopathic physicians as Max Otto Bruker, Karl Otto Heede, and Ralph Bircher.

❧ Fresh Grain Porridge for Sluggish Bowels ☙

2 tablespoonsful of each of the following:
freshly milled grain (the type of grain is a matter of taste,
   and variation is recommended)
whole linseed
ground nuts (any type except peanuts)
finely chopped dried fruits (figs, dates, prunes, raisins, etc.)

Pour enough fresh water over this mixture so that it is completely covered, and allow it to "swell" overnight. If you like, you can add sour milk, kefir, or yogurt before eating the mixture (which should be neither too dry nor too liquid) for breakfast. *Please do not add fresh fruit (despite the illustrations on many cereal boxes), since a combination of grains and fresh fruits will inevitably lead to fermentation dyspepsia and pro-duce distressing symptoms in those who are just beginning to acquaint their stomach and bowels to such a new food.* The diet in general should be adjusted to consist of vegetarian whole foods, and *no further laxa-tives should be taken on any account.* When this fresh-grain porridge is eaten daily for breakfast, it can be guaranteed that within three days a regular stool habit will be set up that is appropriate to the constitution and way of life of the patient. For the transitional phase while one is adapting to the new diet, as Dr. Bruker points out in some of his books, whole grain bread and pastries should not be accompanied by fruit juices, otherwise fermentation will occur in the intestines and cause flatulence.

Linseed: Laxative Without Side Effects

Linseed, the gentle benefactor of the intestinal mucosa, is generally ac-cepted along with wheat bran as being the top healer among swellable fiber and ballast substances. In addition to the fact that it provides plenty of fiber, its oil and mucilages do not merely reduce irritation and heal the damaged intestinal mucosa, but also make the intestinal contents very slippery. *For the treatment of constipation linseed is meant to swell in the intestines, and its increase in volume triggers increased motor activity in the intestinal wall. This is why linseed must be taken whole to combat constipation.* Take one tablespoonful of whole seeds two to three times per day. *It is of great importance that you also drink suffi-cient liquid with the seeds.* It does not matter what you drink, but *you must consume two cups of liquid when you eat whole linseed;* other-wise hard clumps of linseed can build up in your intestines. The recently reported case of a woman who took linseed without sufficient quanti-ties of liquid and almost had to be operated on for complete intestinal blockage emphasizes the importance of this point. It is also crucial to divide the daily total amount of three tablespoonsful into three doses. (Please note the difference when linseed is used for gastric and intestinal inflammations, as discussed on page 160.)

Prunes and Figs

It is also possible to employ soaked prunes and dried figs to combat less severe cases of constipation. After you have soaked the dried fruits over-night in a cup of water, eat up to five next morning on an empty stomach and then drink the water you used to soak them in. If only all medications tasted as delicious as these household remedies!

A Personal Story

Finally, I (Barbara) would like to include my personal experiences with sluggishness of the bowel as a case history. As a young girl I suffered with constipation over a period of years. I tried all the usual medicines and made the equally usual discovery that they were either too weak or too strong in their effects. The situation became worse when I was a student and lived alone, since I began to eat very irregularly and—like many young women—became obsessive about being slim. Whenever I allowed myself to eat anything I prayed that it would not cause me to put on weight, but in fact I oscillated violently between strict abstinence during the week and boundless lust for food on the weekends when I visited my family.

One day it became clear to me how insane and unthankful it was to eat something and at the same time hope that it would not nourish me. With meditation and yoga practices I learned—by no means overnight—to accept and love my body as it was and to treat it with gratitude and affection. I began to cook for myself, to buy organically grown food and have those wonderful mueslis for breakfast, and from then on I never suffered from constipation again in my life. Nowadays, during periods of prolonged traveling, if for some reason my bowels decide to take a day's rest, I forgive them graciously and simply let events take their course without getting nervous about it.

I am relating this story because I know all too well how typical I was then for today's mentality, particularly that of young woman and girls. It is only to be hoped that the highly overrated super-slender ideal for women will finally be rejected in the light of reason and the information now available regarding eating habits. Our digestive systems are responsible for providing nourishment for all the cells of our body. The strength and vitality with which we meet the day, even our thoughts and feelings are dependent upon proper digestion. As we have pointed out, the key is a healthy, natural diet and an active lifestyle.

~ 13 ~

HEALING HERBS FOR PROSTATE, KIDNEYS, AND BLADDER

Most noble, and above all intellectual brilliance, all philosophy and theology, is the readiness of one man to help another—the job of being a brother.
Albert Schweitzer

The phenomenon of prostate hypertrophy in elderly men remains medically unexplained. Why the prostate gland increases in size is unknown, although it is presumed to have something to do with a hormonal imbalance. Nevertheless, it is a fact that 60 percent of men over the age of fifty develop what is known as a prostate adenoma.

PROSTATE SYMPTOMS AND USUAL TREATMENT

Painful symptoms arise because the urethra, the duct located directly below the bladder, becomes narrowed and subjected to continual pressure by the growth of the prostate gland. This causes bladder-emptying difficulties in the form of a constant, painful urge to urinate (which is particularly unpleasant at night) and delays in the start of micturition. The symptoms normally grow worse over the years, so that the bladder loses some of its elasticity and cannot be completely emptied as a result of urine retention and loss of tissue tone. This constant retention leads to chronic irritation and inflammation of the bladder, the ureter, and

179

the prostate itself. The final stage of the disease can be marked by retention of urine in the kidneys and renal insufficiency, which is equivalent to a slow self-poisoning of the body because of the inability to naturally discharge toxic substances. Furthermore, prostate cancer is the third most prevalent form of cancer in men. Therefore, it is important to consult a urological specialist when any of these symptoms occur. He will be able to exclude the possibility of cancer in most cases by means of a simple manual investigation and will normally have no objections to the use of medicinal herbs.

The usual treatment for the disease pattern described above involves the administration of sulfonamides and antibiotics or hormones, which are quite unsuitable for long-term treatment. Even surgical removal of the adenoma often does not completely relieve the painful symptoms, and may be problematical, as is any surgical intervention in the case of older people. Since all these interrelated sufferings are usually chronic in character, the prostate patient is in desperate need of relief by nontoxic medication treatment.

A NEW CURE: SMALL FLOWERED WILLOW-HERB

In this connection, Maria Treben again deserves recognition for having made us all conscious of a valuable medicinal herb that had been long neglected. It is the willow-herb (*Epilobium*), which has more than twenty subspecies. Although it is extremely difficult to distinguish between these subspecies, there are hints that the group of the small flowered willow-herbs (*Epilobium parviflorum, Epilobium palustre, Epilobium alpinum*) are the most effective medicinally.

Willow-herb grows mainly in forest clearings, in quarries, and along roadsides in Europe and North America. It literally multiplies "like a weed" wherever it gains a foothold by means of its prolific, airborne seeds. This is why you should be careful not to let it spread everywhere once you have it in your garden. The herb has also been successfully cultivated for several years, which has shown that harvesting, drying, and cutting are relatively easy. The whole herb is used, except for the roots.

To prepare the tea, two teaspoonsful of dried herb are steeped for four minutes. During the acute stage of adenoma, three to four cups of the tea should be taken daily for four to six weeks, then take two cups daily for several months. If the capsules are taken, the dosage is two capsules three times a day (taken with sufficient liquid) during the acute stage, followed by one capsule three times a day for several subsequent months.

Healing Properties of the Herb

Since the appearance of Maria Treben's book, which has remained in print for many years now, this herb has been employed empirically in thousands of cases and has met with considerable success. Medical scientists have now been forced to direct their attention to this "modern" medicinal herb and finally have begun to investigate it properly. Thus we are pleased to announce the results of a hitherto unpublished West German study that confirms that *Epilobium parviflorum,* in the form of tea or capsules containing the whole herb extract, is an effective yet completely innocuous broad-spectrum medicament for the treatment of prostate adenoma and associated disorders. This medicinal herb, which causes absolutely no side effects, is first and foremost a preventative that each and every man over fifty should take daily. Second, it is an excellent permanent and long-term therapeutic and can serve as a supportive agent in problem-free combination with any other form of prostate treatment, including surgery.

Clinical studies have revealed that teas and aqueous extracts of *Epilobium parviflorum* contain (besides tannins, flavonoids, and triterpene acids) phytosteroids, among which the major active agent is beta-sitosterol. *Epilobium parviflorum* is one of the many plants that contain beta-sitosterol, but it is one of the few to contain it in a medicinally sufficient quantity and usable form.

Small flowered willow-herb tea has been demonstrated to have an inflammation-inhibiting and healing effect on acute and chronic inflammation of the prostate, as well as in the first and second stages of prostate adenoma (there is also a third, or advanced, stage). The annoying symptoms are considerably reduced in a relatively short period of time. It is also effective when employed as a supportive measure following prostate surgery. A real value of this herb also lies in the fact that many patients are spared surgery altogether, because the enlargement of the

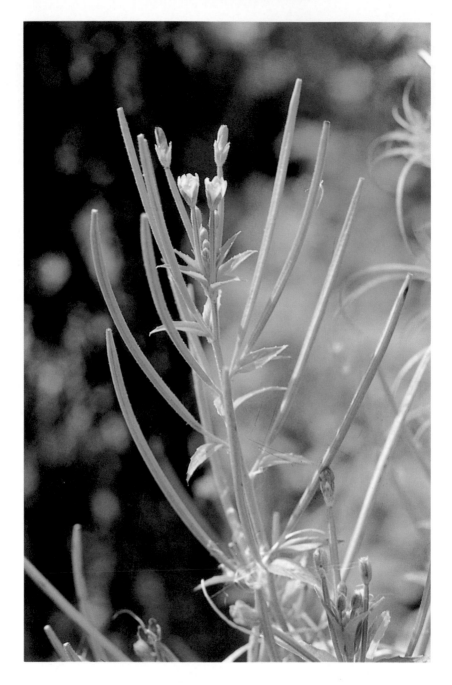

Small Flowered Willow-Herb   *Epilobium angustifolium*

prostate is either significantly slowed down or completely halted. Willow-herb not only is recommended for men but also is indicated for women who suffer from chronically irritated bladder or acute inflammation of the bladder or urethra, since it has an inflammation-inhibiting effect and is a mild and gentle diuretic (a medication that increases urine production).

Ingestion of pumpkin seeds is also recommended to help alleviate the distressing symptoms of prostate disorder. You can prepare them by a gentle roasting in the oven or in a frying pan and season with a pinch of salt or a sprinkling of natural soy sauce, then simply nibble them like nuts.

HERBAL DIURETICS

Flushing out the kidneys and bladder plays a very necessary and important role in natural healing and is in no way restricted to the correction of edema (pathological accumulation of liquid in the tissues). Remember that the urine constantly removes varying concentrations of metabolites, toxins, and other excretory products from the body. Imagine what drastic damage could be inflicted on your health if this purification process were disturbed! This is why diuretic (flushing-out) healing methods have been so successful in such acute and chronic disease states as migraine, asthma, circulatory disorders, rheumatism, and gout.

KIDNEY AND URINARY TRACT INFLAMMATIONS

Inflammatory and bacterial disorders of the kidneys and the lower urinary tract are the major field of application for herbal diuretics. These disorders appear most frequently among pregnant women and older women and can easily become chronic and lead to the so-called irritated bladder. The painful symptoms associated with them are a frequent need to urinate, although with little excretion of urine, a burning sensation and pain in the region of the kidneys, especially when palpated (a sensation often referred to as "back pain"). Sometimes painful spasms are present, and some infections of the urinary tract are even accompanied by fever.

Children can acquire bladder catarrh easily by sitting and playing on wet grass or cold, wet concrete or stones. The danger of a bladder chill is particularly great in the case of young children who may have wet pants or diapers in winter or in cool weather. It is of particular importance here to combat the disorder with the correct measures from the start instead of allowing it to develop over weeks and months until the mass of bacteria spreads to a point where it can only be stopped by antibiotics. When the inflammation has not advanced very far, it is sufficient to increase the amount of urine with an herbal tea in order to aid the urinary tract's self-purification processes and to eliminate invading bacteria (especially coliform bacteria) in a natural manner. Of course, it is a good idea to assist such renal flushing with a general fortification of the immune system by simultaneous application of echinacea tincture.

EFFECTIVE KIDNEY-ACTIVE HERBS

In contrast to chemical preparations, which often cause unphysiological salt losses, most herbal diuretics simply increase the excretion of water and so are ideal for flushing out the kidneys and the urinary tract without causing any imbalance in the body's water equilibrium. Certain herbal preparations lead to increased flow of blood through the kidneys and stimulate the production of what is known as primary urine from tissue fluids, a result that is highly desirable in the case of older people. In addition, the considerable quantities of potassium salts present in various kidney-active herbs lead to water diuresis by osmotic mechanisms; such herbs possess antibacterial and spasmolytic (cramp-relaxing) effects as well.

The following herbs can be combined as desired to prepare herbal teas for flushing therapies to treat the entire urinary tract: birch leaves, dandelion root with herb, bearberry leaves, goldenrod, restharrow, stinging nettle, horsetail, small flowered willow-herb. To ensure success in applying these teas it is essential that at least 1½ to 2 quarts of herbal tea be consumed daily. Six cups per day (equivalent to 1½ quarts) will not be found excessive if they are spread out over the entire day.

Since each one of these medicinal herbs has a somewhat different effect and works on different mechanisms of the body, we recommend blending several of the herbs together. Our standard kidney and bladder tea, with which we have achieved excellent results both with our children and with our adult customers, and which has a relatively pleasant flavor, is blended as follows:

❧ Kidney and Bladder Tea ❧

5 parts birch leaves
4 parts bearberry leaves
3 parts dandelion root with herb
3 parts rose hips with seeds
3 parts goldenrod
2 parts kidney bean pod
½ part hibiscus flowers

This tea should not be consumed over prolonged periods (for more than three months at a time), because bearberry leaves contain high amounts of tannins; neither is it necessary to take it for a longer time to effect a proper cure. Again, please remember that *a flushing-out therapy is not suitable for the clearance of water accumulated in the tissues (edema) as the result of heart or kidney insufficiency.*

Incidentally, it is our opinion that every cancer patient who has had to undergo treatment with cytostatic drugs should drink copious amounts of kidney-bladder tea mixtures to eliminate the toxins and metabolic waste products from his or her body as quickly as possible.

Birch Leaves

The birch tree (*Betula pendula, Betula pubescens*), which grows all over Europe and Asia and in the temperate zones of North America, is one of the most excellent herbal diuretics we have. The young tender leaves must be collected in May and June and air-dried immediately afterward. Used either as a single herb tea or mixed in a formula, birch leaves will increase the amount of urine—both produced and released—and is therefore used in flushing therapies, in cases of inflammatory processes of the urinary tract, and for the prevention of kidney stones. The diuretic effect of birch leaves is mild and nonirritant and so has no detrimental side effects on the kidneys. The infusion from birch leaves should be allowed to steep for ten minutes. Because of its wide assortment of active ingredients (including flavonoids, essential oils, bitter substances, tannins, saponines, and vitamin C) this herb is also used in general cleans-

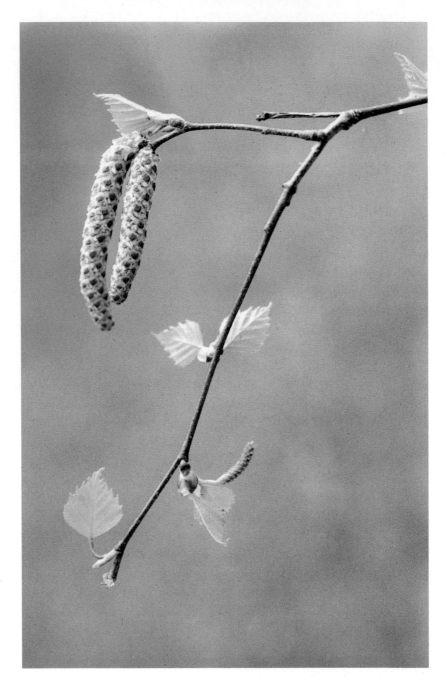

BIRCH LEAVES *Betula pubescens*

ing teas for blood purification, springtime cures, fasting, weight reduction, rheumatism, and so on (see chapter 5 and especially the formula for Blood-Purifying Tea, page 55).

Goldenrod

Goldenrod (*Solidago virgaurea*) is another one of our kidney-bladder herbs. The plant grows up to three feet (one meter) high and can be found on dry grasslands and sunny forest meadows through Europe, Asia, and North America. Its tiny, shiny, golden panicled blossoms appear in late summer and continue to bloom throughout the fall. The plant has a pleasant aromatic smell, yet its taste is hot and very strong. For collecting, the upper part of the plant including the flowers is preferred over the woody lower part. In many gardens, various hearty relatives of medicinal goldenrod are cultivated for their rich golden color.

Goldenrod is used very much the same way as birch leaves for eliminating water retention, for flushing the kidneys and urinary passageways in cases of bacterial infections, and for general cleansing cures. It is also used in tea blends for blemished skin and in rheumatism and gout teas. Also, this herb is effective for the excretion of kidney gravel and the prevention of kidney stones. More than other herbs recommended for urological disorders, goldenrod seems to be the ideal remedy for the kidneys themselves. Clinical studies have shown that it is able to heal both acute and chronic nephritis (kidney inflammation); homeopathy applies it for these conditions as well.

Acute nephritis must not be considered a minor problem, especially when accompanied by high fever and a sudden retention or blockage of urine flow. *In such cases, it is crucial to have a medical doctor ascertain precisely what has caused the inflammation.* If the reason is not any kind of obstruction of the ureter and therefore a backing up of urine, copious amounts of goldenrod tea can effectively help without the risk of any detrimental side effects.

Horsetail Sitz Bath

The effect of herbal tea on acute, painful inflammations of the urinary tract can be supported by a horsetail sitz bath. Since horsetail leaves are relatively hard (see page 49), it is best to soak two or three cups of the fresh or dried herb overnight in three to four quarts of water. Bring to a boil the next day and let the herb extract for ten minutes. Strain off and pour the extract into a sitz bathtub or a normal bathtub and add sufficient water at body temperature to cover the lower back and kidney region, leaving the heart and the chest above the water line (see pages 36–37). You can remain in this wonderfully comfortable bath for ten to fifteen minutes, and the bath may be repeated every other day. It promotes healing considerably.

Chamomile Vapor Bath

Another supportive measure that is particularly acceptable to small children as well as to the elderly is a cramp-relaxing, inflammation-inhibiting chamomile vapor bath for the lower abdomen. As in the case of the chamomile vapor face-bath (see page 77), begin by preparing a chamomile infusion with one cup of chamomile flowers and about one quart of water in a shallow plastic container of suitable size. Place the container down inside the toilet bowl so it rests against the sides of the bowl above the water level and the patient sits directly on it or on the toilet seat (if the seat can be juxtaposed directly over the container itself). Take care that the vapor is not too hot at the start and that the patient does not get burned. This application is capable of relaxing cramps in the region of the kidneys and bladder within a few minutes and is highly appreciated by patients. The same treatment is also very helpful for lower-abdominal pains associated with the start of a woman's period (see page 208).

KIDNEY AND BLADDER STONES

Kidney stones—or more correctly, urolithiasis, the disorder they cause—are another serious problem in the urological field. Every person who has reason to believe that he or she is susceptible to kidney stones, whether by reason of family history, self-observation, symptoms, or medical diagnosis, should regularly drink an herbal tea made from goldenrod, restharrow, and stinging nettle. Naturally, this holds even more true for those who have already suffered acute kidney stone colic, since the rate of recidivity for the disorder is extremely high (on average 60 to 70 percent). Kidney stones are produced when sediments and crystals are formed in the urine and, over the course of years, build up into such

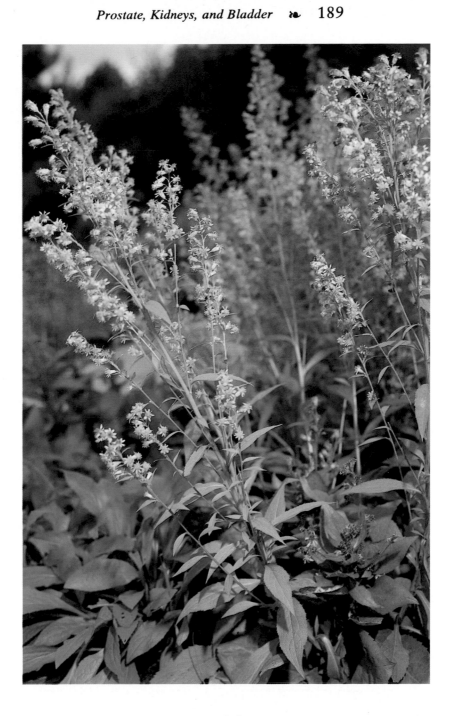

GOLDENROD   *Solidago virgaurea*

large "stonelike" deposits that they block the ureter or urethra if they enter it and give rise to excruciating pain.

The aim, which can be achieved with the aid of the herbs mentioned, is to either stop the growth of kidney and bladder deposits or to flush them out in the form of kidney gravel (particles the size of grains of sand) before they reach the size of "stones" (see also page 51). Even academic medicine has introduced and recognizes a whole range of herbal medicines for long-term prevention of kidney and bladder stones. All these herbal medicinals operate in similar fashion by increasing the dilution of the urine through increased liquid consumption, thus enhancing the dynamics of urine flow. We recommend the following herbal tea for prevention of urinary stones:

&ea; Tea for Prevention of Kidney ∾ and Bladder Stones

5 parts restharrow root
5 parts stinging nettle
5 parts goldenrod
5 parts dandelion root with herb

The medicinal herbs restharrow, stinging nettle, and goldenrod have been proved by medical science to prevent urinary stones and flush out kidney gravel; we believe that dandelion is also indispensable in the same context. This tea produces no unwanted side effects. We advise drinking two to three or—even better—four to six cups daily, since a significant amount of liquid intake is critical for success.

Interestingly enough, it has been demonstrated that our modern diet with its excess calories in the form of protein, fat, and sugar, and its lack of fiber, along with the large quantities of alcohol that are often included, is a major reason for the widespread occurrence of kidney stones. Based on a study of the food consumption of kidney-stone patients, and the concurrent observation that vegetarians rarely suffer from these stones, experiments have been made using bran preparations for kidney stone prevention—with very good results.

FLUSHING TEA FOR RHEUMATISM

To patients who suffer rheumatic pains, we always recommend the following tea as a supportive measure in addition to any other therapy they might undergo.

🙿 Rheumatism Tea 🙿

6 parts stinging nettle leaves
5 parts dandelion root with herb
3 parts birch leaves
3 parts raspberry leaves
2 parts willow bark
1½ parts hibiscus flowers

Take five to six cups of this tea spaced out over the entire day. For best results this dosage should be maintained for a period of three to six months or longer. Such treatment with herbal tea usually does bring relief, but it happens so slowly that patients sometimes do not even realize it!

In this as well as previous formulas, dandelion root and herb appear again and again as an excellent medicinal herb for changing a faulty metabolism, because of its effects on both the liver and the kidneys. (For a more detailed description of this herb, see pages 46–48.)

DIURETIC FOODS

Certain vegetables and fruits increase the flow of urine, a fact that you can observe in your own body. Celery root (celeriac), parsley root, asparagus, and pineapple are examples of such diuretic foods. When it is medicinally appropriate, you should incorporate them into your diet in copious amounts.

❧ 14 ☙

HEALING HERBS FOR WOMEN

Herbs influence both our physical and our spiritual being.

Sun Bear, Chippewa healer

As in the case of nervous disorders and psychogenic headaches (which are discussed in chapters 9 and 10), both mental and emotional factors are fundamentally present in the field of feminine complaints. In today's world, where men and women work together on an equal footing, there is little place for the natural rhythmic processes that spring from the female being and little freedom to live by the alternating phases of expansion and retreat. For the woman of today there is often a severe tension between the requirements of work and career and the needs and wants of creating a harmonious family life, and this tension makes itself well known on the physical level. (See the book *The Second Shift,* by Arlie Hochschild and Anne Machung [New York, 1989].) Not surprisingly, woman's attitudes toward sexuality, partnership, and motherhood also play a decisive role in disorders of the sexual and reproductive organs. However, inasmuch as gynecology deals with organic diseases, their diagnosis and treatment must be left to the medical specialist. If a complaint lasts for longer than one week you should consult a gynecologist. Please allow yourself to be examined and together with the doctor try to reveal the cause of the problem. *Only when you leave the doctor's office knowing that there is nothing wrong organically, that the disorder is what medical practitioners describe as an "autonomic nervous disorder," is it appropriate for you to treat yourself. The consequences of not following this important rule can be disastrous.*

Medicinal herbs are ideal for the treatment of autonomic imbalance of the reproductive organs and for complaints during menopause. They can gently and harmoniously compensate without interfering harshly in the complex and subtle hormonal processes that direct the equilibrium of the female body.

Autonomic nervous disorder predominantly takes the form of diffuse, periodically returning pains ranging from severe cramps to back pain and various types of menstrual disturbances, such as periods that are too heavy, too slight, delayed, irregular, or painful. During practical consultations we have found that the following six herbs have proved themselves useful in relieving such symptoms: yarrow, chamomile, lady's mantle, shepherd's purse, dead nettle, and cowslip. Each of these medicinal herbs possesses a unique and different emphasis and effect, and our experience is that it is essential that the correct choice be made with each individual patient on a case-by-case basis. This can only be done by personal contact and conversation with the patient. For this reason, we will discuss what these six most important herbs can mean for you in order to give some direction as to how to discover the optimal herbal treatment for your condition, or that of a friend, relative, or acquaintance. (Be prepared to find that it will be most difficult to make judgments concerning yourself.)

We are aware that this chapter differs somewhat from the others with respect to the method by which we consider the various indications and remedies. It is perhaps more inspirational and more closely related to emotional, mental, or, if you will, spiritual conditions. We do not have a precise explanation of why this is so, except to say that our perspective has developed over a long period of time from an intense and loving attention to such disorders and to women of all types and constitutions.

YARROW

The number one herb for the effective treatment of a variety of female

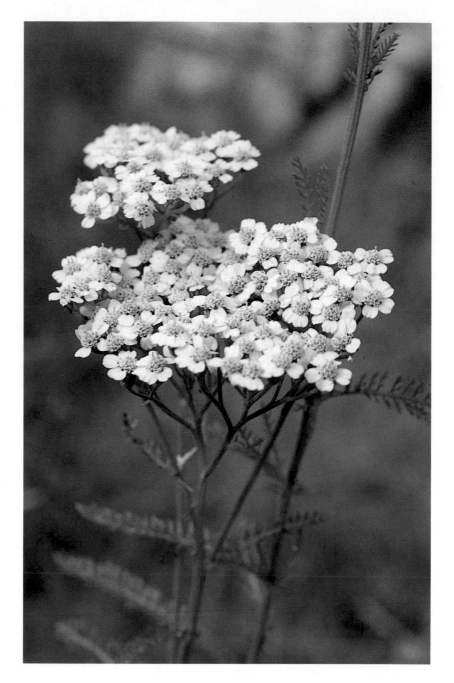

YARROW   *Achillea millefolium*

ills is yarrow (*Achillea millefolium*). This very common, almost inde-structible plant is native to Europe, North America, and northern Asia. It has acquired such diverse names in folk medicines as Achilles herb, bellyache herb, and maiden herb. Its tiny white flowers are tightly packed in an umbrellalike flower head that serves as a favorite dwelling place for insects of all kinds. The leaves are finely pinnate and exude a char-acteristic bitter odor when they are rubbed between the fingers. When you first smell this, you will understand *why yarrow can cause an aller-gic reaction in very sensitive people* who touch it in the wild or use it as a medicinal herb.

Yarrow grows on poor meadowlands, heaths, and embankments and in dry clearings. It is characterized as a steppe plant (a plant of the plains) both by the wiry resistant nature of its stalks, leaves, and flowers and by its hearty resistance to dry conditions of soil and climate. Its constituent ingredients have been thoroughly investigated by medical science: evidently the components of yarrow produce their complex and well-established healing effects only when kept together in natural com-bination, not isolated or separated from each other.

Yarrow's main field of application is for disorders of the stomach and bowels (inflammation, diarrhea, flatulence, and cramps), in which cases it has inflammation-inhibiting, bacterial, antiflatulent, digestion-promoting, and spasmolytic effects. Yarrow is also effective when applied externally in the form of compresses, rinses, or baths, as a wound-heal-ing, inflammation-combating aid for disorders of the skin and mucosa. (See formulas for Stomach Tea 2 on page 158, Liver and Bile Tea on pages 165–166, Wind-Releasing Tea for Adults on page 172, and yarrow bath and tea for infants on page 173.) In traditional folk medicine, yarrow also finds use for treatment of women's complaints, for stanching bleeding, and for menstrual problems, particularly spasmodic periods and prob-lems related to menopause. Yarrow is suitable for tough, resistant women who keep quiet about their disorders and tend to belittle rather than dramatize them. These are women who carry on in spite of the pain and will only complain when things have deteriorated to their very worst.

CHAMOMILE

Chamomile (*Matricaria chamomilla, Chamomilla recutita*), or German chamomile (as it is often called), is perhaps the best known of all medici-

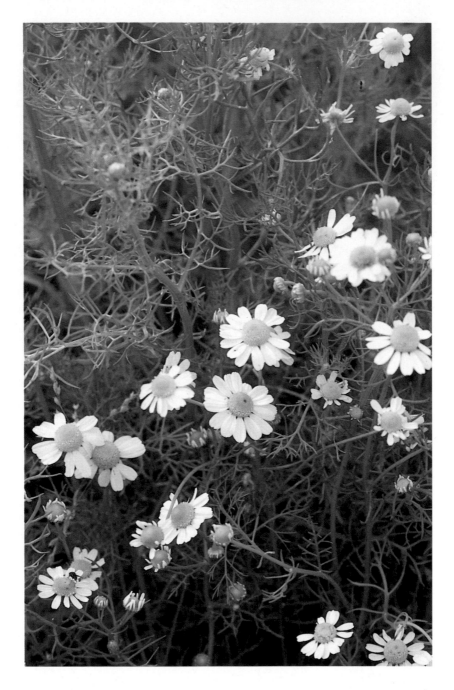

CHAMOMILE *Matricaria chamomilla*

nal herbs. It is manifold and most comprehensive in its healing effects, which can be beneficially exploited by both internal and external applications. Chamomile is a very modest "weed" that grows almost everywhere in Europe, the United States, and Australia, on arable lands, grain fields, fallow land, and dry clearings. It will not, however, grow on land that has been heavily fertilized. Most of the chamomile employed in medicine today is cultivated.

Identifying the Correct Species

When collecting chamomile for yourself from May through June, you must be able to properly distinguish between the true medicinal, so-called German chamomile, the so-called dog chamomile, the rayless, and the scentless chamomile. With the exception of the very rare rayless chamomile, the only true test is to cut vertically through a blossom; in the real healing chamomile, the center of the head will be hollow, while in the other, nonhealing species it is solid. The flowers must be harvested at the right time and dried correctly to gain the optimum yield of their vital, active ingredients. Like yarrow, chamomile has been subjected to rigorous scientific investigation, and clinical confirmation of its effects has been excellent. Among the plant's many components the essential oil, and in particular the chamazulene and alpha-bisalbolol that the oil contains, are the major active substances. When isolated, this essential oil has a distinctive blue color.

The traditional names given to chamomile—mother herb and maiden herb—clearly reflect the fact that the primary use of this healing herb is for women's disorders. In addition, chamomile is the herb of choice for healing skin and mucosal disorders—particularly inflammations—wherever they appear. This is why chamomile is so often used in wound-healing ointments, skin care products, cosmetics, soaps, and infant care products. When it is taken internally, its primary effects are anti-inflammatory and antiflatulent in character. It is of great effect for the treatment of stomach disorders, gastritis, and gastric ulcers (see pages 157, 159, and the following passage). Chamomile in the form of baths, douches, and vapor baths has been found to produce excellent healing effects with inflammations and irritations in the anal and vaginal regions. Chamomile vapor baths in particular are most effective for gynecological inflammations, because the herb's rich essential oils readily volatilize into the vapor of a steam/vapor treatment. This method of

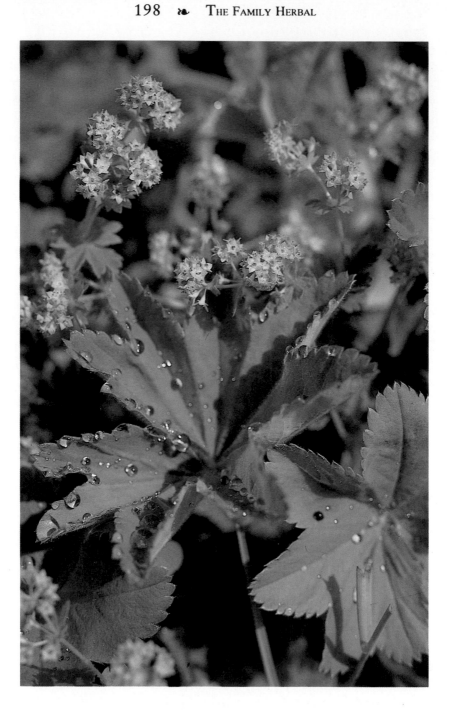

LADY'S MANTLE   *Alchemilla vulgaris*

application also brings out chamomile's spasm-relaxing effect, which can be exploited advantageously during menstrual spasms (see also page 209) and for the treatment of kidney and bladder inflammations (see page 188).

The character of chamomile is best described as being gently loosening and mildly relaxing. In spite of its gentleness, it can, like yarrow, kill off certain fungi and render certain bacterial toxins harmless. However, even the mild chamomile can induce an allergic reaction in people who are highly sensitive to plants of the composite family (Compositae), and with internal applications overdoses should be avoided. In connection with female disorders, chamomile is most suitable for women who tend to be touchy, sensitive, or timid. In particular, young girls who are irritated by and have fear of their monthly periods respond very well to chamomile, as do women who fear their own sexuality yet have great need for tenderness and security.

LADY'S MANTLE

Lady's mantle (*Alchemilla vulgaris*) is another recommendable medicinal herb for female disorders. In our view, this plant enhances the feminine aspect of motherliness. Although scientists remain skeptical about its use in the absence of experimental investigations, traditional medicine has always employed lady's mantle, and in our own experience it has been of assistance in many cases.

Whenever we went collecting lady's mantle our children always derived great pleasure from this herb, which nestles in the thick grass of mountain pastures. The center of the plant's deeply folded leaves often contains a single drop of dew that is held by the silky hairs of the leaf's surface and gleams like a precious pearl. We used to tell our children that the dwarfs drank their morning fill from these enchanting little vessels, and the children delightedly did the same. Some folk stories about herbs say that the drop of water held by lady's mantle is the tear of an elf. One scientific view claims that the drop is not dew but an excretion of the plant containing a high concentration of its active ingredients. The tiny flowers, of an unobtrusive, light green color, form delicate yet dense clusters. The herb blooms from May through September and can be harvested (albeit laboriously) during the entire period. Lady's mantle grows throughout Europe, North America, and Asia.

Scientists are ready to admit that lady's mantle is able to provide an astringent effect against diarrhea and bleeding on account of its high tannin content. Folk medicine further advises that this herb invigorates the female sexual organs, particularly the uterus, and hence is useful in preparation for pregnancy and as a pre- and postnatal aid. In spite of its modest size, this little plant exhibits great strength and power. It is ideal for young women who devote themselves lovingly to motherhood, or at least wish to do so. It is associated with the qualities of gentleness, elegance, and grace, in combination with powerful authority. If a woman finds difficulty in accepting a maternal role, is troubled by thoughts of abortion, and suffers from morning sickness and other disorders during the first months of pregnancy, depression after birth, and so on, then lady's mantle is her herb. It is also appropriate for the mothers of adult children who have identified themselves far too much with their role as mothers, find it difficult to enjoy their new maturity and independence, and now have to go through a reverse process of "leaving" motherhood.

SHEPHERD'S PURSE

Shepherd's purse (*Capsella bursa-pastoris*) has a great deal in common with lady's mantle. Again, scientists put a question mark next to this herb, even though it has established itself as a blood-stanching agent (uterine bleeding) and as a particularly effective aid in the case of excessive periods. Hippocrates is known to have employed shepherd's purse as a medication for the uterus.

Shepherd's purse is another "weed" that grows virtually throughout the world and always follows in people's footsteps. Like willowherb and plantain, shepherd's purse is one of the first plants to colonize bare ground in fields and along paths and even thrives between pavestones and along sidewalks. The herb acquired its remarkable name from the appearance of its fruit, a heart-shaped, tightly packed purse with a seam down the middle. The leaves form a rosette close to the ground and only appear individually farther up the stem. The whitish flowers are tiny and unobtrusive. The plant bears buds, flowers, and fruit simultaneously from spring until autumn.

Shepherd's purse poses unique difficulties when it comes to scientific investigation. It is often afflicted by a white mold that alters its

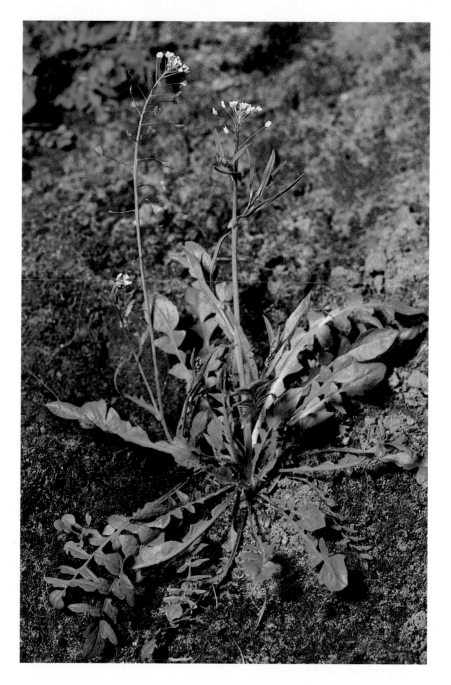

SHEPHERD'S PURSE   *Capsella bursa-pastoris*

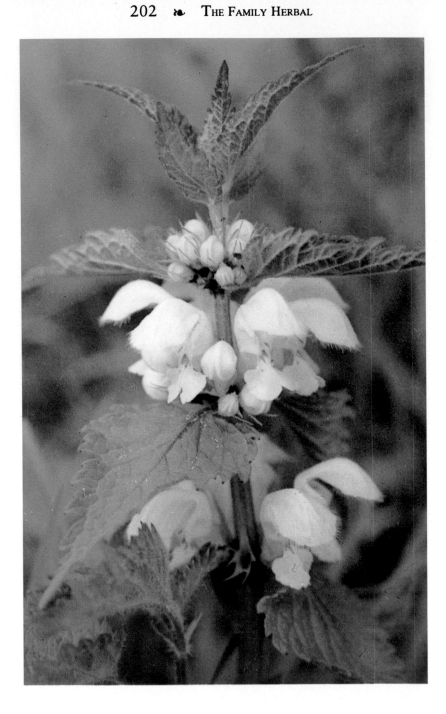

DEAD NETTLE *Lamium album*

naturally occurring substances. The problem is that the mold can be seen only in its advanced state, yet its impact on the plant organism begins long before that time. On the other hand, it is quite conceivable that the mold itself may actually produce the plant's medicinal effect or at least contribute considerably to it. The wide variations observed in the concentration levels of its active ingredients also make analysis of the plant difficult, for these levels vary significantly with the season, weather conditions, and growth site. (For references about shepherd's purse as a medication for high blood pressure, see also pages 144–145.)

We agree fully with the traditions of folk medicine as to the use of shepherd's purse for female disorders, and recommend it for menstrual periods that are too heavy or painful and as a general tonic for the reproductive organs. When the floor of the pelvis, the ligaments holding the uterus, or the muscles of the uterus itself lose tone and elasticity, shepherd's purse tea or tincture can be of good assistance. This is especially true for women whose reproductive organs are exhausted or whose entire body or mental resistance is fatigued, sometimes because of too many or too frequent pregnancies or long periods of unrelieved round-the-clock care of babies and small children. Shepherd's purse women are basically uncomplicated, optimistic, vivacious, and capable of unexpectedly rapid recovery. Use of shepherd's purse can even help them recover quickly from states of complete exhaustion.

DEAD NETTLE

The next herb, dead nettle (*Lamium album, Lamium luteum*), also comes from the rich tradition of folk medicine. It is the white or yellow dead nettle that is most frequently used medicinally, and in general only the labiated flowers are employed. The name is derived from the similarity of this plant's leaves to those of the stinging nettle, the major difference being that dead nettle's leaves do not sting. Dead nettle grows throughout Europe and Asia and likes most to grow in the shade of taller plants such as trees and bushes, particularly in gardens, along the edge of paths, and against fences or walls. It prefers a cool, moist climate. When you collect dead nettle you must take care to distinguish it properly from a whole variety of other plants with similar labiated flowers. Dead nettle's characteristic bittersweet odor can be a key to its identification.

When we were children we loved to pull out the dead nettle flowers and suck them for the tiny bit of sweet nectar they contained. Hildegard of Bingen had a high opinion of the "bee suck," as she called dead nettle. The substances it contains have yet to be properly defined. The herb is used as a cough medicament that promotes expectoration and calms irritated mucosa. In the case of women's complaints, the main indications are irregular and painful periods, inflammations of the female organs, and vaginal discharges. Here the external application in the form of baths can be highly recommended as well. A tea made from dead nettle and sweetened with honey, maple syrup, or rice syrup has a calming and harmonizing effect. The dead nettle type is a woman with a harmonious nature who feels happy and completely at ease with her life. She is feminine and sensitive, and also steadfast and self-confident. In fact, just about everything is fine for her—if only she didn't have these symptoms.

COWSLIP

The last plant on our list is cowslip (*Primula veris*). This tiny, sweet-smelling spring flower with hanging yellow blossoms hides in grasses and bogs. Its common German name means "heaven's key," a title evidently inspired by the joy of seeing this herald of spring at Eastertime. It grows in Asia and Europe and favors the lower slopes of the Alps, sunny meadows, and sparse bush country, preferring the banks of brooks and streams. It is found almost exclusively in March and April. Its existence has been threatened by the use of artificial fertilizers, which is why it is a protected species in Germany. *Those who are allergic to the whole genus of* Primula *should not use cowslip.*

The roots of the cowslip are used for coughs on account of their saponin content (see the formula for Cough Tea 2, pages 80 and 86). Folk medicine also attributes to it curative powers in cases of neuralgia, migraine, and problems related to menstruation and menopause. Cowslip flowers are of particular help to tense, intellectual women who tend to react hysterically, whose emotions vary greatly, and who are affected by changes in weather and often suffer from headaches or migraine attacks (see chapter 10). We have observed that cowslip is especially effective when such headaches regularly occur along with the monthly period and are often accompanied by dizziness and a rush of

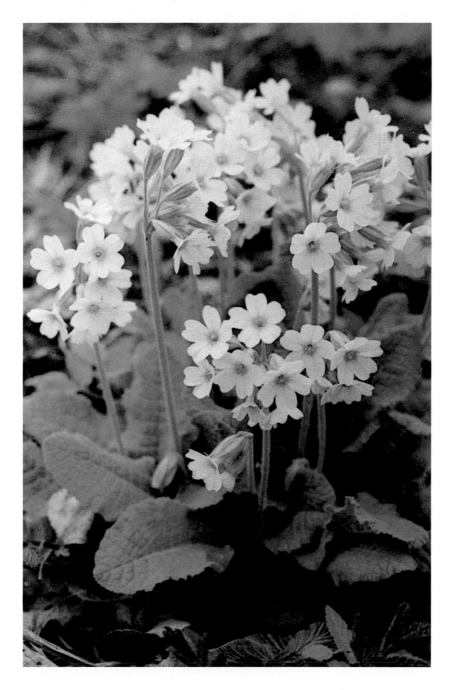

Cowslip *Primula veris*

blood to the head. This form of premenstrual syndrome can be significantly improved by long-term treatment with cowslip flower tea. This is also true when such symptoms occur at the change of life. Cowslip, with its characteristic qualities of freshness, innocence, delicacy, and subtlety, is able to bring the easily high-strung woman back to her natural equilibrium.

CHOOSE THE HERB THAT'S RIGHT FOR YOU

The six "feminine herbs" we have described can be taken alone or in combination as tea blends. From the descriptions given, choose the herb that feels right for you. Their effectivity can even be increased when they are taken as herbal tinctures. The following basic tea can be employed as a start for treatment.

⚬ Basic Female Tea ⚬

6 parts yarrow
6 parts lady's mantle
4 parts chamomile flowers
4 parts shepherd's purse

The other two "feminine herbs," as well as herbs for other indications, can be added to this blend to create your own special formulation. A good suggestion would be to add herbs for nerve-strengthening, calming, or vitalizing. Here are some examples: if a patient is anxious, add 6 parts balm leaves; if she tends to depressive moods, add 6 parts St. Johnswort; if she is pregnant, due to deliver shortly, or has just given birth, increase the proportion of shepherd's purse to 10 parts or add another 2 parts of dead nettle; if she has hot flashes relating to menopause, then add 6 parts cowslip. The appropriate blend needs to be taken not merely when complaints appear, but in a dosage of two to three cups daily for several weeks, in order for the full potency of the herbs to take effect.

The following tea blend tastes most pleasant and brings balance to women whether they are suffering from symptoms or not:

⚬ Woman's Tea ⚬

5 parts lady's mantle
3 parts yarrow
2 parts elder flowers

2 parts chamomile flowers
2 parts hibiscus flowers
2 parts rose petals
1 part shepherd's purse
1 part black cohosh root
1 part raspberry leaves
1 part peppermint leaves
½ part cornflowers

FOR EXCESSIVELY HEAVY PERIODS

When your periods are too heavy, it is advantageous to take fifteen drops of shepherd's purse tincture three times per day, in addition to drinking one of the above-mentioned tea mixtures, over a period of several weeks. The dose can later be taken just three to four days before the period is due to begin each month, but only after considerable improvement has been observed.

In addition, be certain to supplement your intake of assimilable iron. Everyone knows that in our bloodstream iron acts like a magnet, attracting and carrying oxygen throughout our bodies. With the multitude of denaturalized foods of today, our iron reserves (stored in the liver) can easily be depleted by excessive menstrual bleeding, pregnancy, breastfeeding, or times of extra stress, resulting in fatigue and lack of vitality. Iron supplementation is of course a must for patients with anemia. To effectively replenish any iron deficiency, you must know a few things: The best absorbable form of iron is iron-II-lactate, which is better tolerated by the stomach than iron gluconate. It also reduces the known side effect of iron preparations, constipation, because the lactate releases the iron molecules gradually into the blood. The absorption of iron is definitely inhibited when milk, coffee, or black tea is consumed, and considerably enhanced when vitamin C is present. That's why it makes a lot of sense to combine iron with fruit and vegetable juices or concentrates from red beets, black currants, carrots, and spinach. Maximum absorption is also aided by taking the iron preparation before meals. For an herbalist, a thought that suggests itself is to combine the iron lactate with a special selection of herbs that in themselves provide iron in organic composition. Such a selection would include stinging nettle, yarrow, lady's mantle, and shepherd's purse, supported by gentian, bitter orange peel, garden sage, rosemary, and balm.

MENSTRUAL CRAMPS

Nothing is better than a yarrow bath or sitz bath for treating cramps at the start of a period. These acute convulsions can sometimes even lead to circulatory collapse, for which we offer an herbal medication on page 148. Prepare this bath by pouring one to two quarts of boiling water over a handful of yarrow herb, leave covered to steep for twenty minutes, then strain off. Add this extract to a normal full bath; half the quantity is sufficient for a sitz bath. Our experience is that these cramps always disappear completely within ten to fifteen minutes of such bathing. They can even be completely prevented by taking the bath before you feel your period is about to begin and before the cramps begin. If you learn to handle your menstrual problems in this way you will never need to use chemical painkillers for ordinary cramps. If the pain does not subside, or bleeding becomes heavier, discontinue the bath and seek medical attention to find out whether you have a fibroid tumor, endometriosis, or some other disorder.

Chamomile Vapor Bath

A chamomile vapor bath can also be effective against menstrual cramps (see pages 188 and 197 and the illustration on page 77 for details on how to prepare the bath). If you are not in a position to prepare an herbal bath or vapor bath, it is often helpful to simply take a normal hot bath for fifteen minutes or to place a hot water bottle on the lower abdomen for about half an hour. To prevent menstrual cramps we also recommend that in addition to your individually blended herbal tea or the Basic Female Tea (page 206) you take yarrow tincture regularly for several weeks: fifteen drops, three times per day.

PREMENSTRUAL SYNDROME

The so-called premenstrual syndrome, which includes such symptoms as tension, painful and sensitive breasts, nervousness, irritation, sleeplessness, headache, and loss of performance and productivity, can be treated in the same fashion as other female complaints. Take a tea from the six "feminine herbs," plus yarrow tincture (ten drops, three times per day) and in addition, a weekly bath either with yarrow alone, or with yarrow and lady's mantle, or with yarrow and dead nettle.

As a personal remark in this connection, we would like to say the following: It seems to us that in the United States, in recent years, almost too much attention has been directed toward symptoms of premenstrual syndrome, thus providing both women and men with good reason to play them out and dramatize them even more. In our opinion, a slightly noticeable energy drop, a bit of tiredness the night before, and a slight tension in the breasts are nothing to worry about, nothing to avoid, and not associated with disease or malfunction. I (Barbara), as a woman, must admit that my attitude toward menstruation in general has changed quite a bit since my participation in a women's seminar with an American Indian mentor. This teacher made me understand that this "lack of performance" is not necessarily a bad thing! The fact that we have slowed down and may be a bit less companionable is the very thing we must appreciate. The urge to withdraw, be by ourselves, retreat, and reflect during those special days is our great chance and challenge to be a woman in the fullest sense—be sensitive, be open, feel and listen. So let us be grateful that Nature herself forces us into a passive, contemplative mood once every month; this is just what the world needs.

Vaginal Discharges

Vaginal discharges are best aided by sitz baths with yarrow, dead nettle, and lady's mantle (mixed or used separately), but only when your doctor has established that it is not a fungal or bacterial infection.

When the outer and inner sexual organs are inflamed, what is appropriate is heat treatment in combination with herbs. Here again, the chamomile vapor bath has proven particularly effective (see the discussion on page 188). In this case the vapor bath can also be made with equal parts of yarrow and chamomile. It is important to always keep the lower abdomen, legs, and feet warm if you are susceptible to such inflammations.

Problems of Menopause

Hot flashes, outbreaks of perspiration, nocturnal sweating, nervousness, irritability, headache, sleeplessness, fatigue, mental strain and tension, a low feeling, a sense of lost performance—these are all typical symptoms of menopause. They can be considerably ameliorated by an individually blended mixture of the six "feminine herbs," of which cowslip flowers must be the major element. One cup of this tea each morning and evening is the minimum requirement. The flavor can be varied by altering the blend slightly week by week. This tea will also support medical treatment by a doctor if that becomes necessary. When the symptoms of menopause are that the woman feels nervous and cannot come to terms with herself, we recommend the following tea mixture:

❧ Menopause Tea for Nervous Women ❧

6 parts balm leaves
4 parts St. Johnswort
4 parts hop cones
4 parts lady's mantle
4 parts cowslip flowers

FASTING CAN HELP

We have been told by many of our women friends and patients who have gone through the change of life that the hormonal adjustment can be far more easily mastered when a fasting cure is taken once or twice a year. (Fasting is discussed more extensively in chapter 5.) This again shows that the freer of pollution and toxins the organism is, the more able it will be to react to specific conditions and demands and to balance itself.

HELP FOR EXCESSIVE PERSPIRATION

The annoying symptom of outbreaks of perspiration that is often experienced during menopause can be ameliorated with sage tea. The tea must be prepared very strong to help diminish excess perspiration. Place three teaspoonful of sage leaves in a saucepan and add two cups of boiling water. Cover with a lid and simmer for five minutes. Drink two cups per day of this tea, either hot or cold. This dosage is not recommended for people with sensitive stomachs. You can read more about sage in chapter 7 (pages 87–89).

PREPARING FOR CHILDBIRTH

Now, a word concerning childbirth. We recommend taking lady's mantle tincture (ten drops, three times a day) beginning four weeks before the baby is due. The same purpose can be fulfilled by drinking two cups of lady's mantle tea three times a day. Every expectant mother should in addition take ten drops of homeopathic arnica 5x, three times daily, beginning ten days before the expected delivery date.

All three of our children came into the world by natural childbirth and were delivered at home. The use of St. Johnswort oil was an extraordinary help, and we are glad to share our experience with you. During the birth and in the last stages of the delivery, the midwife liberally lubricated the vaginal walls with St. Johnswort oil, to aid the delivery of the baby's head. As soon as the birth was complete, St. Johnswort oil was applied to the vulva to promote rapid healing and tissue regeneration. We have also used St. Johnswort oil for the care of the newborn. After his or her first bath, we applied it over the baby's entire body, taking great care to reach every little skin crease, yet *not* to take off the vernix caseosa, the whitish substance found in the newborn's skin creases.

LYING-IN

There is no better beverage than herbal tea for the period of "lying-in" and the initial weeks and months of breast feeding. You can alter the flavor as you desire, and you'll be providing your body with life-giving healing forces dissolved in lots of liquid without any calories! Also remember that herbal teas contain vitamins and minerals as well.

If a nursing mother is not producing sufficient milk, a special tea can be of great help. Here's the recipe:

🌿 Lactation Tea 🌿

4 parts anise seed
4 parts caraway seed
4 parts dill fruit
4 parts fennel seed
4 parts vervain wort (blue vervain)

Since this tea consists almost entirely of a mixture of closed, hard seeds, they should be crushed before brewing. This can be done manually in a mortar or in a kitchen mill or blender in the same manner as nuts or coffee beans are ground. You have to make this extra effort, since virtually none of the active ingredients will be extracted from the seeds by simply brewing it. (See also page 170.) But please, crush only as much as you are going to consume immediately for making the tea; otherwise you will lose the active ingredients that are mainly contained in the essential oils and the aromas. The herbs are brewed into a tea in the normal manner and allowed to steep for five to ten minutes. As a general rule in breastfeeding you should recognize that it is the amount of fluid the mother consumes daily that is the decisive factor in milk production.

The subtle, complex nature of a woman's system is perfectly suited to the subtle, complex character and action of medicinal herbs. As in all matters of health, the key to restoring and maintaining a woman's health naturally is a combination of personal responsibility and preventative care.

❧ 15 ☙

*HEALING HERBS
FOR FIRST AID*

> *All things are poison and nothing is without poi-
> son. It is the dosage alone that makes a thing poi-
> sonous or not.*
>
> Paracelsus

ARNICA

An herb that can truly be called the first-aid plant of natural medicine
is arnica. Compared to the host of often very unassuming medicinal herbs,
arnica is a most imposing plant personality, not just because it is extremely rare and because where it does occur its brilliant golden-yellow
flowers turn the mountain meadows into a living carpet of exploding
color, but also because of its unmistakable aromatic fragrance and its
powerful medicinal effect. *Arnica is so strong that it can cause severe
toxic symptoms if incorrectly administered.* For this reason, the saying
of the master physician and alchemist Paracelsus that serves as the epigraph to this chapter is especially applicable to this precious healing plant.
"All things are poison and nothing is without poison. It is the dosage
alone that makes a thing poisonous or not." We would add that it depends upon the method of application as well—as we can also learn by
studying Paracelsus's medical writings.

The medicinal herb *Arnica montana* is a plant that grows almost
exclusively in mountain regions, at heights from 2,400 to 7,500 feet (1800
to 2500 meters) on rugged, turf-covered meadows and isolated,

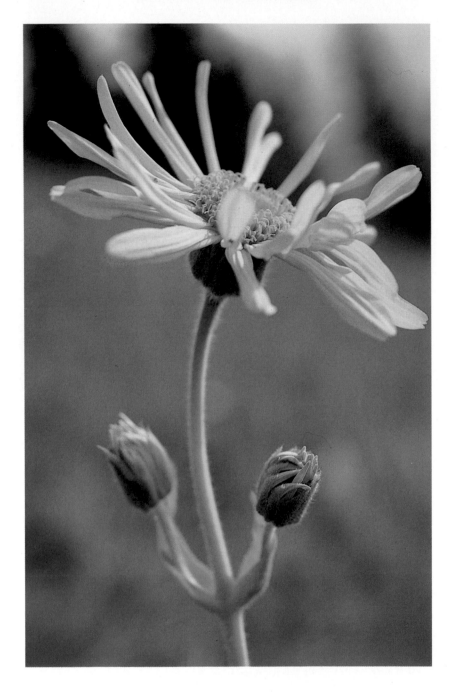

ARNICA   *Arnica montana*

unfertilized pastures. It thrives solely on lime-free, acid soil and in a cold, moist climate. A German folk name for arnica literally means "mountain well-being." The plant blooms between June and August (depending on the height at which it is found). Usually only the flowering head of the plant is collected for the preparation of arnica tincture. The rootstock is employed for homeopathic preparations.

We must earnestly advise that you *do not collect arnica yourself,* not only because in many places the plant is protected and would become even more depleted by unauthorized uprooting, but also because many other yellow-bloomed Compositae with which arnica can quite easily be confused grow in the same alpine meadows. In addition, it is necessary to make sure when harvesting the flower heads that none containing the larvae of the arnica fly are collected. Nor is there any need, in fact, to go to the effort of locating the herb yourself: every herbalist and natural food store herb section should have arnica tincture and homeopathic preparations of proven quality.

The European immigrants to America made arnica known in the new world, and for a long time they imported it from Europe for lack of their own domestic supply. After many years the native arnica species were tested for effectivity and included in the American Pharmacopoeia. One species, *Arnica chamissonis,* was found to be as effective as *Arnica montana* but had the distinct advantage that it was much easier to cultivate. This variety was then reintroduced into Europe and since that time has been cultivated for medical purposes, especially in eastern Europe.

As is true in the case of many Compositae, there can be allergic reactions toward arnica; it is mainly pale-skinned redheads and blondes who cannot tolerate it and who tend to react with skin problems even when arnica is applied in the proper dilution. Fortunately, however, anyone who is aware that such sensitivity is present or who cautiously tries out the tincture on a small patch of skin and reacts adversely can turn to comfrey instead, since various indications for the external application of the two plants coincide.

Do Not Use Arnica Internally

Internally taken, arnica affects the heart and circulation, where the correct dose is the crucial issue. *If too high a dose of arnica is taken internally, massive intoxication can occur, and the subsequent irritation of the intestinal mucosa can cause vomiting, diarrhea, and bleeding. In addition, dizziness, trembling, heart racing, irregular pulse, and breathing difficulties can occur. Extreme cases of massive overdose can result in circulatory collapse and respiratory spasm leading to respiratory failure.* For these reasons, *we advise principally against taking arnica internally* for heart problems, particularly since there are other medicinal herbs which can be used to treat the heart effectively but with much less risk. However, *it can be taken with no risk at all in homeopathic dilutions and preparations,* and we would not want to forgo arnica's astonishing effectivity in this type of preparation.

External Use of Arnica

The many active components of arnica ensure that its effects when externally applied are very wide-ranging. It has disinfectant, antiseptic, and antifungal properties and promotes wound healing. The main area of application for arnica is the external treatment of all types of injuries in which the skin is not broken, such as bruises, pulled muscles and tendons, contusions, hemorrhages, and swellings, including those related to bone fractures. The speed with which the correctly diluted tincture has healed such injuries has astonished us time and time again. In one such case a friend of ours received a very painful bruise on the wrist while roller skating. An arnica compress reduced the pain and swelling to a minimum within twelve hours, and the joint was almost back to normal within three days. As you may know, such injuries can occur frequently during sports, particularly in team games where the play can be very rough, when skiing, or in falling from a horse or off a bicycle as well as in such extreme instances as automobile accidents. In your own home or at work similar mishaps can occur, like falling off a ladder or falling down the stairs. In such instances, the most important thing is to *apply an arnica tincture compress immediately* or as soon as you possibly can. The following two points must be taken into account as well.

1. *The compress should never be applied to an open wound* but should only be applied where the skin is whole and intact. (Although arnica can be an excellent wound-healing agent, the tincture would cause unnecessary burning to an open wound, because of its alcohol content.)
2. When you purchase arnica tincture it is usually between 120 and 160

proof. *This concentrated arnica tincture must never be applied right from the bottle,* but diluted (1 part tincture to 5 parts water) before use.

Arnica Compress

To prepare a compress, measure out a tablespoonful of arnica tincture and five tablespoonsful of water into a bowl or cup and mix them (see figure 11.) Double both qantities if you need to cover a very large area. Dip a piece of cotton (of a size appropriate for the affected area) into the liquid; wring it out over the bowl so that it is moist but not dripping wet, and lay it on or around the injured part of the body. Then apply a light piece of cotton cloth and cover with a light bandage only to keep the compress in place. When the cotton has dried out, you can moisten it again with the tincture-water mixture simply by applying it through the bandage, so that the dressing does not have to be removed.

Our Personal Experience

Even though we have been spared severe injuries, we can recount from our own experience dozens of family situations when arnica tincture came to the rescue in a time of acute need. One day, during our elder daughter's gymnastics lesson, a heavy bar was inadvertently dragged over the foot of one of her schoolmates. Although the child cried dreadfully and her foot turned red and blue and swelled badly, the teacher apparently did not recognize the severity of the injury and took no action. Our daughter had with her an arnica pad (a damp paper tissue soaked in diluted arnica tincture, something like the refreshing moist travel pads one can buy). She placed the pad on her classmate's foot, and the pain died down immediately. By the end of class, the swelling had subsided so much that the child was able to put her shoe on and walk home!

Once, during a camping trip in America, the car door was slammed on the finger of our youngest child. The skin was unbroken, so we bound it with an arnica pad (which we never travel without). The finger did not swell at all, and the pain quickly ceased. Luckily there was no fracture, and within a few hours after applying the pad we were able to forget all about an incident that could have been much, much worse. We still remember with pleasure the lasting impression this treatment made on our American friends who experienced it along with us.

Another time, one of us was taking part in a yoga course and strained

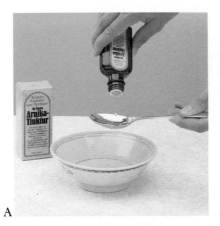

A

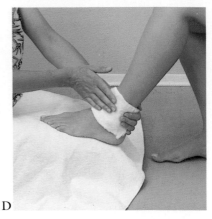

D

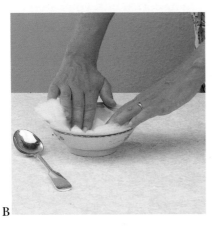

B

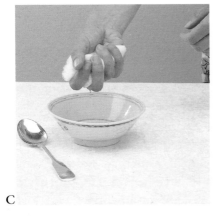

C

Figure 11

Arnica Compress

A. Measure one tablespoon of arnica tincture and five tablespoons of cold water into a shallow bowl.

B. Dip a piece of cotton into the liquid.

C. Squeeze out slightly.

D. Place the moist cotton on the painful or swollen area.

E. Cover with a piece of light cotton cloth and secure with a light bandage.

F. To renew the compress, moisten the cotton again by applying the tincture-water mixture through the bandage without removing the dressing.

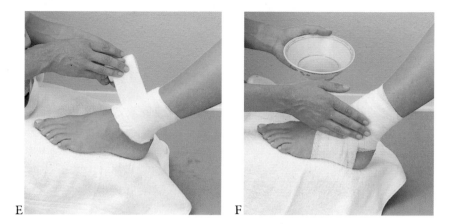

E   F

a tendon in the foot by sitting in the lotus posture far too long. Two days of rest from the exercises and several repeated applications of arnica compresses, and all was well again.

Finally, we will never forget the recurring shock of seeing our son at ages two, three, and four years falling and banging his head on stone steps, the edges of walls, and the corners of seemingly every piece of furniture in our home. Each time we would watch as an enormous bump grew on his head within a few minutes. An arnica compress was applied as quickly as possible on each occasion, and we would watch the bump subside and disappear almost as quickly as it had come—within about ten minutes! We have personally observed instances in which swelling and the red or blue bump (effusion) that follows such injuries did not even form when an arnica compress was placed on the affected area within the first minute or two. As a consequence, the pain too was reduced very rapidly. If you keep this extraordinary herbal remedy close at hand and therefore can act soon enough, more often than not it will quickly seem as if the injury had never occurred at all!

Homeopathic Use

After every type of shock or trauma, the injured person should receive Arnica 5x or 10x. Homeopathic drops of arnica are also an aid in coping with a situation when the shock is of a mental character. The administration of Arnica 5x once or twice daily for seven to ten days before an operation is scheduled will help promote rapid postsurgical healing without complications. It can also be taken before childbirth with similar results (see page 211).

In homeopathy as well as in herbology, arnica is considered one of the most important and effective medications for accidents, injuries, and situations of shock. Numerous homeopaths have reported rapid reduction of pain and quick healing with the administration of Arnica 5x or 10x in the case of bone fractures, painful luxations, contusions, concussion, and open wounds resulting from accidents. In German, arnica is called "the fall herb," which reflects its long history as the external and homeopathic internal treatment of choice for falls, spills, and other injuries.

Arnica Ointment

As we have already noted, arnica ointment is particularly useful for the long-term follow-up treatment of bruises, strains, sprains, contusions, and effusions, and as a postsurgical application for bones, tendons, joints, and muscles. It also works quite well as a healing ointment for wounds, grazes, scratches, and many types of skin eruptions. It disinfects insect bites and reduces itching. In cases of blemished skin and acne, arnica cream has proven to be very helpful as well. (See also pages 55–56.)

Combining Various Applications

In order to experience for yourself just how remarkable arnica is, and to know we have not exaggerated in the least, please try the following recommendation. The compress is the first measure for all the injuries we have described. The second step is the administration of homeopathic Arnica 5x tincture. (Please be certain you understand the difference between a regular tincture and a homeopathic tincture by referring to the passage on tinctures on pages 38–39.) The third step is the renewing of the compress, which may if necessary be kept on and remoistened periodically for a period of days. Finally, the application of arnica ointment is an ideal fourth step when the compress is removed, as it contains arnica tincture (although in lower concentration). The combination of externally applied arnica tincture and the internally taken homeopathic preparation strongly increases the resorption of effusions of blood in bruised tissue.

THE GENTLE POWER OF CALENDULA

If arnica is the first-aid herb for injuries in which the skin is not broken, calendula is its counterpart for open wounds. In our opinion, any natural home pharmacy cannot be without it, particularly if there are children in the family.

Marigold, or pot marigold, is a pretty and decorative garden flower that grows in bright sunny places without being too fussy about soil conditions. Its big brilliant yellow or orange composite flowers and luxuriant greenery add a vigorous splash of color to nearly every park and garden. For centuries it has been part of the standard palette of every traditional cottage garden.

Since many people use the folk name *marigold* to refer to a number of totally different plants (e.g., *Tagetes*), we prefer to use its Latin name, calendula (*Calendula officinalis*), to avoid such confusion. Calendula is a generous and uncomplicated plant that blooms throughout the entire summer from May to October until the first frost. It is presumed that this property led to the plant's being given the Latin name *calendula,* for the Romans, who were certainly acquainted with this wonderful medicinal, used to call the first day of each new month *calends*. Calendula was widely used in the Middle Ages: the great healer Hildegard of Bingen (1099–1179) used it to treat impetigo and skin blemishes, Albertus Magnus (1193–1280) praised its effects as a healing agent, and it is described as a reliable wound healer in the famous herbal *Hortus sanitatis* (1485) and in numerous later herb texts. This characteristic was confirmed by Father Sebastian Kneipp (1821–1897), who recommended the plant for varicose veins, bedsores, and skin blemishes of all types.

Calendula is native to the Mediterranean region and today is cultivated there on a large scale for medicinal purposes. Either the whole flower blossom is employed or the petals alone without the calyx. Extensive research programs conducted recently at universities in Germany and Italy have extended our knowledge about the combination of effective compounds in calendula, i.e., triterpene alcohols, carotenoids, flavonoids, and triterpene glucosides, among which the main active ingredient is faradiol ester. The flower's bright yellow-to-orange color is due to its extremely high content of carotenoids, a substance of great importance for all the bodily functions, particularly eyesight and the ability of the skin to regenerate itself. Carotenoids are relatively stable chemical

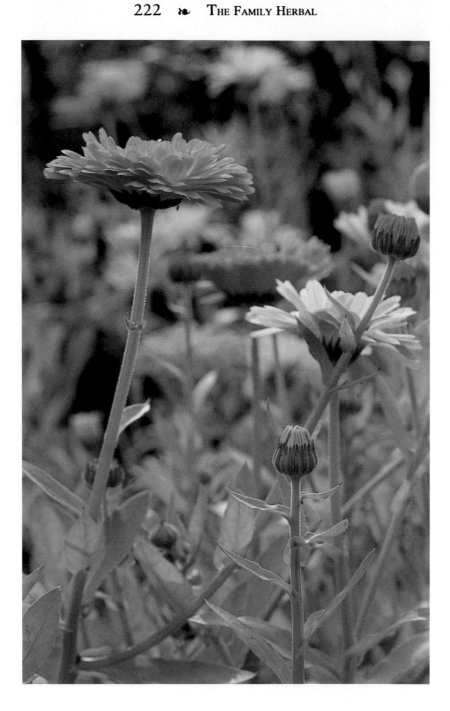

CALENDULA   *Calendula officinalis*

compounds that are soluble not in water but in fats. This factor helps to determine what medium is selected for extraction when preparations are made from calendula.

CALENDULA TEA

In principle, calendula can be employed in the form of a tea, decoction for compresses and douches, tincture, oil, and ointment; depending on the extraction medium used, different substances will go into solution. In fact calendula is rarely employed in tea, except as a decorative herb to make colorless herb mixtures more attractive (for example, see page 176). However, calendula tea is not without effect. It has a spasmolytic, bile-stimulating, and blood-purifying effect, which gives good reason to include it into a stomach or bile tea. It can also be used to good effect in women's tea for treating menstrual pains.

CALENDULA INFUSION FOR EXTERNAL USE

A monograph on herbal medicinal substances presented in 1987 by the German Bundesgesundheitsamt (Federal Health Authority) confirms that calendula flower petals have an inhibiting effect on inflammatory processes in the mucosa of the mouth and throat and that an infusion of calendula has a healing effect on cracks, bruises, and burns. In fact, compresses or douches with calendula infusion promote tissue granulation in fresh wounds as well as in chronic, poorly healing wounds, leg ulcers, and local dermal inflammations. The treatment is carried out by preparing an infusion with one handful of calendula flowers to one quart of water, and then proceeding exactly as described for horsetail (see pages 51–52 with accompanying illustrations). Calendula tincture can be employed in exactly the same manner. For a mouthwash or a woundhealing compress, use two teaspoonful of tincture in one cup of water.

Calendula flowers are a frequent ingredient in cosmetic ointments, face lotions, regenerating skin ointments, hair care products, and soaps on account of the plant's ability to care for the skin and to heal damaged epidermis. Calendula oil is especially suitable for the care of infants and for adults with very sensitive skin.

HOMEMADE CALENDULA OIL

If you have many marigold (calendula) plants in your garden you can prepare calendula oil yourself. To do this, place freshly harvested but quite dry flower heads loosely in a transparent, wide-mouthed glass jar and add cold-pressed vegetable oil to cover. Seal the jar so that it is airtight and leave it for four to eight weeks, shaking vigorously once a day. When the oil has acquired a deep yellow color, press out the flowers. Filter the oil through a sieve and store it in a dark bottle. This ready-to-use skin care oil can be kept for at least one year.

CALENDULA OINTMENT

The calendula preparation that is employed most, and which is the most convincing in its effect, is the ointment. It has a long tradition and in earlier times it was prepared in every farmhouse across the land for treating domestic animals as well as for the family's personal use.

Calendula ointment was once traditionally made using lard. The lard played two vital roles: first, as an extraction agent—since carotenoids are soluble in fats—and second as an ointment base or carrier. Tradition also holds that lard itself can act as an antibiotic ointment. In our own pharmacy we still have an antique apothecary jar labeled "Adeps suillus" ("pig lard"). We have found that lard is an excellent carrier substance because of the close similarity of its fat cells to those found in human skin. Lard therefore enables the extracted active substances of the herb to penetrate through the levels of the skin down to the areas where they are needed most. However, because many people have a distinct aversion to lard and cannot tolerate the idea of putting it on their skin, we have also found alternative ointment bases consisting of vegetable oils and beeswax.

In this context we must also mention the modern technology of extracting fat-soluble ingredients in medicinal and food plants by the help of carbon dioxide (CO_2). Unlike the hitherto customary extraction media for lipophil substances—chloroform, benzine, acetone, and ether—all of which are somewhat toxic and leave residues in the processed plant material, the gas CO_2 has all possible advantages on its side: it is a completely natural substance obtained directly from the earth from volcanic wells (you may know that carbon dioxide is what makes still mineral water sparkle). It is 100 percent pure and abso-lutely unpoisonous. It does not leave any residues whatsoever in the extract. It is not harmful to the environment and can be recycled and reused (in other words, the same portion of gas used for one round of extraction can do the job several times). Last but not least, CO_2 is the best and most thorough solvent of all. Admittedly, however, the in-dustrial machinery needed to apply such a so-called "super-critical gas" is very complicated, huge, and expensive, since the procedure has to be carried out under certain conditions of pressure and temperature during which the gas is transformed into a liquid and then retrans-formed into a gas. All marigold products produced by Naturwaren (in the United States, NatureWorks) contain concentrated extracts obtained through this technical procedure. At Naturwaren we have conducted research to define the active ingredients in calendula flow-ers. The goal of that research has been reached, and the results have been published in the book *Die Ringelblume* by Otto Isaac (Stuttgart: Wissenschaftliche Verlagsgesellschaft, 1992). For the consumer this means that marigold creams and salves made by NatureWorks are now standardized products for which we guarantee equal potency and effectiveness at all times, even though they are plant medicinals. For the community of professional herbalists, the definition of the main active ingredient now leads to the next step of breeding new botanical varieties that will contain a maximum quantity of the main active in-gredient.

Benefits of Calendula Ointment

Calendula ointment is an exceedingly versatile and excellent medica-ment for treating wounds, burns, skin problems, venous congestion, varicose veins, and decubitus ulcers (bedsores), this last condition a widely encountered problem in bedridden patients. It has been clearly demonstrated in all the above conditions that calendula ointment accelerates the healing of both large and small wounds, promotes granulation of tissues, and inhibits inflammatory processes, because it is bactericidal toward staphylococci and streptococci. The ointment also stimulates the supply of blood to the skin, making it more supple and hence more resistant to mechanical and chemical irritants. It rap-idly soothes the pain and is extremely easy to apply, and there are no restrictions whatsoever to its use on account of tolerability or unwanted side effects.

Calendula ointment can especially be recommended for poorly healing chronic wounds such as leg ulcers, which often occur in the elderly as a result of poor blood supply to the extremities plus venous insufficiency. The ointment also promises success for abscesses, running sores, and purulent wounds.

Our Personal Experience with Calendula Ointment

We wholeheartedly recommend calendula ointment and use it in our own family whenever a wound needs to be treated. It gives us rapid relief when it is applied to cracks, contusions, and scrapes as well as burns and scalds. The ointment successfully inhibits infection of the wound with its attendant inflammation and suppuration. Indeed, we cannot remember a single instance of any such complication occurring after a wound was treated with calendula ointment.

Apart from the numerous minor scrapes and bruises that we have treated successfully in ourselves and our children with calendula ointment, two cases in our experience were particularly impressive. One involved Peter's brother Siegfried, who was severely wounded on the lower leg as the result of a motorcycle accident. The wound simply did not heal for weeks. Only when the shiny red, suppurating wound was coated several times a day with calendula ointment and dressed freshly each time did signs of healing begin. Remarkably enough, the wound healed over within two weeks. On our advice, it was then continually treated in the same way for a longer period. Later, the scar was massaged with calendula ointment as well. Today, there is no sign of a scar. We have observed these results—the smooth and soft healing of scar tissue following injury or operation—in many other instances as well.

The second case was that of a woman who had undergone radiation therapy for a cancerous growth on her neck, leaving a patch the size of the palm of your hand where the skin had simply disappeared and the raw flesh was exposed. We recommended compresses of calendula infusion twice a day and continual application of the ointment. The hideous-looking wound healed over smoothly in a relatively short period of time. Overjoyed, as you can well imagine, the patient visited us one day and showed us her perfectly recovered neck.

HEALING THE SKIN

Small cracks in the skin, such as the splits, chapping, and fissures that often occur on the lips, in the corners of the eyelids, on fingers, or on the nipples, can often be very painful. These heal quickly if they are massaged with calendula ointment. The ointment can also be a help in all types of bacterial or fungal infections of the skin around the mouth or in the region of the anus, for locally limited itching eruptions such as diaper rash, and even for athlete's foot. It is true that in cases of allergic outbreaks and other exanthema, calendula does not remove the internal causes (e.g., immune control disorders, metabolic disorders, or nerve irritation), but it can ameliorate the patient's acute feeling of skin tension or itching and shorten the duration and clearing time of skin eruptions.

As mentioned above, the carotenoids in calendula ointment act to restore the skin's own powers of recovery. For instance, calendula ointment is perfect for hands that have become rough, chapped, and cracked by extended contact with harsh detergents, soap powders, or other chemicals, or when the face or lips become rough and raw through exposure to extremes of weather. The daughter of one of our friends had painfully sore and swollen lips caused by the cold last winter. She tried calendula ointment on our advice after her usual lip salves and ointments had brought no relief, and achieved very rapid results.

We always recommend calendula ointment as an indispensable skin protection when applying a Swedish Bitters compress (see pages 104–107). If it should ever happen that you develop an allergic reaction to an herb or a skin irritation is caused by the application of an herbal compress, then calendula ointment is the remedy of choice.

For us, the most convincing evidence of the efficacy of calendula as a skin ointment was presented when our younger daughter, Maria, was a baby and often had a sore bottom. The reddened skin sometimes gave her so much pain that it was impossible even to touch it, never mind to wash her. A single application of the soft, fatty ointment usually did the job, so that by the next morning the redness and soreness had always disappeared as if by magic. The diaper rash that newborn infants and often older babies suffer from wearing disposable diapers is also rapidly cured in this way. We know of nothing better than calendula ointment and calendula oil for baby care and for the gentle care of irritated skin. We also have several men friends with sensitive skin who use calendula as a soothing aftershave ointment.

Whenever we attend meetings and trade fairs (which we do several times a year), along with all the other participants we suffer from dreadfully heavy, aching feet and often painful pressure spots and abrasions. After a warm footbath and a short plunge in cold water, we like to massage calendula ointment into our feet. Every time, we find that they are refreshed and fully recovered by the next morning.

VARICOSE VEINS

The problem of varicose veins is statistically more likely to affect women than men; the main causes of this condition are overweight, too much sitting, and too little exercise. The particular pressure relationships upon the major pelvic veins during pregnancy and the extreme burden placed on the legs in the final months of term frequently trigger the first painful symptoms even in younger women. Long periods of standing every day can also have a similar effect, particularly when there is an inherited trait for vein and tissue weakness.

For persons with such predispositions it can be of utter importance to prevent problems by early supplementation with silica. In the human body, silica—in a colloidal (gel-like) form—plays an active role in giving tissues body, firmness, and strength, as well as in bone formation and remineralization. Extensive studies in the United States, Germany, and the former Soviet Union have shown that as we age our supply of silica is increasingly depleted, resulting in wrinkled, dry skin; dull, lackluster hair; and brittle nails. When such signs are observed in a patient, one can be sure that the bone structure and connective tissue are in dire need of silica and that the probability of venous deficiencies and complaints is very high. Silica, acting as a binding agent, enhances the body's ability to increase the water absorption of essential proteins. By binding existing calcium, protein, and water molecules together, they help to retighten connective tissue and remineralize bones. Although in the world of herbs horsetail offers a very high content of silica (see page 49), extensive clinical studies have shown that silica in a colloidal gel form is even better absorbed.

Varicose veins and venous congestion occur when larger or smaller leg veins lose their tone and elasticity and greatly increase in diameter. This means that the venous valves, which work as one-way valves like floodgates or locks, no longer close properly and sufficient blood is not pumped toward the heart. Instead, the blood remains in the legs, the tissue fluids become overloaded or congested, the blood thickens because its flow rate is diminished, and eventually the poorly supplied tissue tends to become inflamed. The more this condition deteriorates, the greater the danger of thrombosis and embolism. Because of these possible complications *a doctor should always be consulted for advanced varicose veins or for phlebitis,* which can become very painful. The first signs of these disorders are swelling of the foot joint (edema), great sensitivity of the skin to pressure (such as from wearing garters or elastic-topped stockings), and—above all—a heavy, tense, hot sensation in the legs that becomes especially bad when the temperature climbs. Calendula ointment is very effective for relieving these symptoms. The legs should be rubbed regularly with the ointment mornings and evenings. We recommend also that you wear elastic support stockings if you suffer from this problem.

In the initial stages of venous complaints, natural stimulation such as treading water, walking in grass wet with dew, or cold rinses can be most helpful in preventing further deterioration in the tone of the veins. But the most important thing is sufficient exercise taken regularly (e.g., walking, jogging, or dancing). After work or outdoor activity, the legs should be showered from the knee down (first with warm water, then with cold) and rubbed with calendula ointment; the feet should then be elevated for a period of rest.

In all cases of venous inflammation the ointment should be applied very liberally and, if possible, covered by a light bandage. To keep it on for a long time—if possible, overnight—is a factor of particular importance, since it allows the medicinal or healing substances of the herb to penetrate most deeply. When applied consistently, calendula ointment greatly decreases the symptoms of varicose veins, venous congestion, and phlebitis by inhibiting inflammation and, at the same time, by tautening the tissues and promoting enhanced blood supply to them. These effects have been reported by many of our patients and customers, and we have been able to observe the course of treatment very closely in the case of one of our grandmothers. Besides supplementing the diet with silica gel, it is generally advisable to accompany this treatment with a diuretic tea in order to stimulate the excretion of water, the need for which is indicated by the appearance of edema in the feet and lower legs. Our tea blends for kidney and bladder (pages 185 and 190), Rheumatism Tea (page 191), Slimming Tea (page 59), and Blood-Purifying Tea (page 55) are all equally suitable for this purpose.

HEMORRHOIDS

Like varicose veins, the complaint of hemorrhoids (which affects 25 percent of adults at one time or another) is also caused by a general weakness of the venous blood vessels. Here too, pregnancy is often the triggering factor in women, since the fetus exerts a strong pressure on the major pelvic veins in the last months of pregnancy. Again, we recommend calendula ointment, especially when the painful or itching hemorrhoids are close to the anal opening and hence can be treated without difficulty. The presence of bleeding or painful hemorrhoids is good reason to ensure that the stools are very soft. For this purpose, refer to the Laxative Tea given on page 176 (and please be sure to read our caution there).

BEDSORES

We recently discovered a new field of application for calendula ointment, with which we had had no direct experience ourselves, namely decubitus ulcers (bedsores), or pressure sores. Sister Birgit, an intensive-care nurse at a large hospital in Munich, who was very interested in natural healing and herbal recipes, introduced the regular treatment of calendula ointment for the bedridden patients in her department. She and her colleagues observed that this measure brought about a dramatic decrease in the number of cases of bedsores. Sister Birgit's enthusiasm for calendula ointment reached other departments in her hospital and even other hospitals, and eventually clinical studies were made in several hospitals and old people's homes. The result was a clear endorsement of calendula as an eminently well-suited ointment for the effective prevention of bedsores.

From Sister Birgit and the nursing staff in Munich we learned that pressure sores are an enormous and almost intractable problem in intensive care units and facilities that care for older people. Whenever people are unable to move their bodies, there is a real danger that the skin at the typical contact points of the body (the back of the head, the shoulders, the base of the spine, and the heels) will suffer from an inadequate flow of blood and become sore. The constant pressure at these sites over a period of a few hours or days is enough to damage the skin, and once open sores have appeared they are exceptionally difficult to heal. The patient often suffers great pain and discomfort, and the condition of the skin at this stage requires a tremendous amount of additional nursing effort.

It was certainly in the best interests of the nursing staff to test the effects of calendula ointment, especially as few of the existing ointments, powders, air cushions, or plasters had produced any satisfactory results. Tests over several months revealed that patients whose problem areas were rubbed twice a day with calendula ointment according to our prescription very rarely developed bedsores. The rich quality of the ointment was expressly praised by both nurses and patients alike. The brittle, cracked skin of most of the affected elderly patients was made soft and supple again by the calendula ointment, unlike other available preparations, which were too rapidly and superficially absorbed. The observed increase in blood supply meant that it was no longer necessary to apply alcohol-containing skin friction rubs to promote blood flow, a distinct advantage since these rubs also have a pronounced drying effect on the skin. In conclusion, we recommend to all doctors, nurses, and lay people who have to care for immobile or bedridden patients that they try calendula ointment as a prevention against bedsores. As always, an ounce of prevention is worth many pounds of cure.

16

AN HERB FOR ENERGY AND VITALITY

O mickle is the powerful grace that lies
In plants, herbs, stones, and their true qualities.
For naught so vile that on the earth doth live
But to the earth some special good doth give.

William Shakespeare, *Romeo and Juliet*

Human beings all through history have searched for the "universal medicine," the "elixir of life," or the "miracle drug of rejuvenation." In the true sense of the word such an herb or drug does not exist; yet, a few medicinal plants exhibit an amazingly broad spectrum of action. The most important and most thoroughtly investigated of these is ginseng (*Panax schinseng* C. A. Meyer). A folk name for this plant in German is "all-heal root," the word "jin-shen" or "gen-chen" in Chinese means "man plant," Korean names call it "life root" and "man root," and the Japanese words "mind-sin" or "nind-sin" translate into "best of plants" or "wonder of the universe." Whereas ginseng has been known as a prophylactic against old-age and disease for thousands of years in Asia, where it is even considered a panacea (derived from the name of the all-healing Greek goddess) and constitutes an intrinsic part of Asian culture, it has been known in the West for only a relatively short time. Ginseng has been shrouded in an aura of myth because of its "exotic origin" and has somehow experienced the same fate as acupuncture, which, though used for thousands of years in the East, was ignored and viewed as ineffective hocus-pocus

232

by the medical profession of the West for a long time just because Western science did not have thought concepts that would accommodate this healing method. Only when many Western physicians and scientists went to China to take a closer look did they acknowledge that acupuncture actually works. In the end they even adopted the concepts of energy centers, flows, and lines through the human body. Finally, when expenditure on acupuncture treatment became tax-deductible in the United States in 1973, the situation all of a sudden changed, and acupuncture became an established technique. Equally, in the decades-long discussion about ginseng, the community of Western scientists did not accept the positive reports until the development of new methods of analysis (such as gas chromatography) and new methods of identification of chemical structures (such as mass spectrometry and nuclear magnetic resonance spectrometry), which made it possible to define the mystery of the pharmacologically active ginseng components.

HISTORY OF GINSENG

This plant's history turns out to be a truly fascinating story, leading back into antiquity. Ginseng was mentioned in the first Chinese treatise on medicine more than 2,000 years ago. According to the legend, the gift of the miraculous root was brought to humankind by an omnipotent mountain spirit in the form of a man-like root, which only the wise and worthy were able to find. Even to the present day, ginseng is considered in Asia to be the royal gift for those who seek a long, healthy, and happy life. A Chinese medical text dating back to 300 C.E. cites ginseng for the preparation of "love potions," in the Liang dynasty (502–555) the plant and its harvesting were described, and in the T'ang dynasty (618–905) it was called a "royal plant." Around 1,000, ginseng root was first brought to Spain by a Moorish seafarer, in 1294 it sailed westward with Marco Polo, and in 1610 it eventually came to Europe once more with a Dutch seafarer. In 1697 its scientific discussion began at the Academy of Sciences in Paris, and at about the same time the Japanese succeeded in cultivating ginseng.

In 1720, the American (specifically, Canadian) ginseng was discovered as a "medicine" long used for various diseases by indigenous Indians. At that time a veritable storm broke out over ginseng. The plant was found growing in the wild and was exported to Canton at ten times

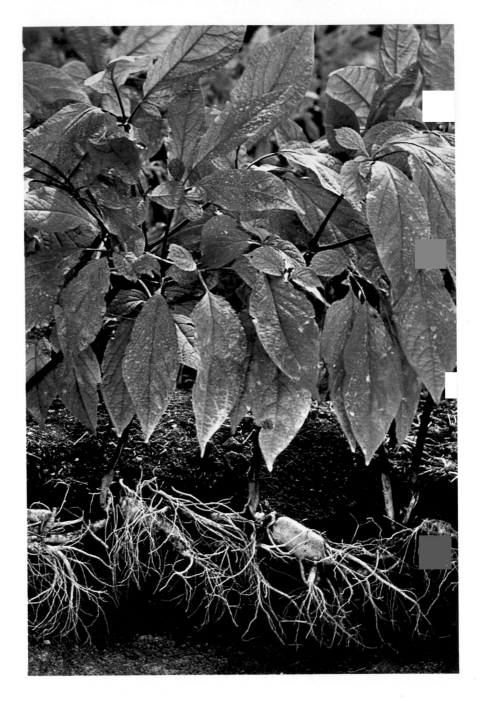

GINSENG   *Panax schinseng*

the price. Although the Canadian ginseng proved to be less effective than the Chinese, massive trade developed between East and West, resulting inevitably in the complete extinction of the wild plant in Canada some 170 years later. At the royal court of Louis XIV, the French Sun-King, the aristocrats fell prey to "Ginseng madness," and in Holland, famous physicians applied the root for treating states of exhaustion and for restoring strength after illness. In the middle of the 18th century, almost every European apothecary stored a ginseng root, even if as a rarity, while the Koreans finally succeeded in cultivating the root. Since China could not continuously produce enough ginseng for its own supply, hundreds of tons of American ginseng were sold to Hong Kong and Canton. In 1842, the German botanist C. A. Meyer designated the Korean ginseng and *Panax schinseng* C. A. Meyer, the species that is today internationally recognized as being the best. In 1902, ginseng root was, according to Mr. Rublee, the American consul general in Hong Kong, an indispensable part of the life of well-to-do Chinese. In the 1920s, cultivation in America was at its peak, centered mainly in Minnesota but also conducted in Wisconsin, Michigan, and Ohio. Only after World War II, when the Soviets occupied Korea, did the Russians become interested in Ginseng root and start their own cultivation. Since 1960, extensive research has been done in European laboratories, particularly in Switzerland and Germany, and many clinical trials have been carried out. One of the aims of the ongoing research today is to win a place in the most important pharmacopoeias for the ginseng extract that has been developed and standardized.

BOTANICAL DATA

Ginseng belongs to the Araliaceae family, like ivy, and is an upright shrub reaching a height of 60 to 70 cm (about 2 feet). The leaves stand in groups of four or five; the fruits are light red berries; the matured root is 10 to 20 cm (4 to 8 inches) long and 1 to 2 cm (⅜ – ¾ inch) in diameter. Besides the Korean ginseng, there are also Japanese, Chinese, Indian, American, and Canadian varieties (*Panax japonicum, P. quinquefolium, P. trifolium, P. repens,* and *P. pseudoginseng*). It has been demonstrated that *Panax schinseng* C. A. Meyer, cultivated especially in South Korea, is pharmacologically the most important. As all who study ginseng are aware, South Korean farmers possess the greatest expert knowledge of ginseng cultivation, acquired through centuries of experience and their readiness to implement the latest biological principles of cultivation for medicinal plants.

The ginseng plant demands a relatively rough climate; however, the air temperature throughout the year must remain between 0 and 25 degrees Celsius. Also, a special type of soil is necessary, and the ground temperature must be as constant as possible. The plants do not tolerate any artificial fertilizer (good for us!) but utilize only a fertilizer made of gathered ginseng leaves, nor can they bear direct sun exposure. For this reason, as we have personally seen in Korea, ginseng cultures are always protected by specially constructed sheds. Although the plants can grow for more than 20 years, only 4- to 6-year-old roots should be harvested in September and October, since they contain the optimal quantity of active ingredients. Their shape is similar to that of a turnip and is frequently compared to that of a human body; their color is brownish white.

As is well known on the market, a distinction is drawn between "white" and "red" ginseng root and preparations. The difference arises from the processing subsequent to harvesting and cleansing the root. What is offered and sold as "red ginseng" is a root that has been subjected to a sterilization process with hot steam, during which the color turns brownish red. White ginseng roots have been carefully sun-dried and therefore do not change their color.

CONTENT AND PREPARATION

As the main active ingredients of ginseng, several glycosides with saponine character have been identified and called ginsenosides. The chemical structures of six main and nine secondary ginsenosides have so far been established. There are also beta-sitosterine, essential oil, panaxacid, estrogen-like compounds, trace elements, and other ingredients. Very important for the health-seeking consumer are the proven facts that ginseng has no allergic or other undesirable side effects whatsoever, that it is not habit-forming or addictive even when taken for a prolonged period, and that it is absolutely safe for human use.

Ginseng root can be eaten (as a vegetable, which is customary in Korea in almost every main course and vegetable dish) or prepared as a tea from the dried, small-cut root. The form usually used, however, is a tincture, specifically, an extract obtained through sophisticated extracting procedures. In the purchase of a particular product or brand, more than with any other herb it is of utmost importance to choose carefully, from among the countless ginseng preparations offered on the market, a standardized product of superior quality. The proper dose of the standardized extract from true Korean ginseng root is 100 mg twice a day for the average adult. Bear in mind that only after regular intake for about four weeks can the full impact of such a "tonic" be felt. Sometimes ginseng extracts are also applied as spagyric essence (5 drops 5 times per day) or homeopathic mother-tincture (5 to 10 drops 5 times per day).

The pharmacological action of ginseng preparations has been described as a so-called adaptogenic effect, which means that it helps the organism to overcome and equalize (balance) harmful influences of all kinds by stimulating the body's own powers of adaptation. It is especially effective for symptoms of stress, such as fatigue, states of weakness and exhaustion, listlessness, nervousness, reduced power of concentration, and slow reaction times. Whether stress is physical or mental, ginseng is truly the right herb to deal with it. Whatever the reason for reduced efficiency or lack of performance may be—emotional problems, a recent illness, menopause, or premature aging—this tonic and energy stimulator can make the difference.

Athletes around the world praise ginseng's tonic action, knowing that although it furthers top performance, it has no doping effect. It does not mobilize the last bit of energy reserves only to leave the person completely exhausted afterward; on the contrary, its action is harmonizing and constructive. Special tests with athletes have demonstated that under physical stress they achieve better performance with ginseng through increased intake of oxygen into the blood and a lowering of the lactate level in the muscles. In this way, the time required for energy regeneration is shortened. World-class athletes should use it; they most certainly would be much better off with such a plant preparation than with doping chemicals. In convalescence, a ginseng preparation helps the person regain natural strength; there, too, it shortens the recovery period.

Various complaints of old age are also benefited by ginseng root. The stimulating effect of the ginsenosides upon the transmitter substances in the central nervous system and the heightened oxygen level in the blood both result in better functioning of the brain, higher mental alertness, improved concentration, and a better memory. If you observe in your grandfather or grandmother those typical signs of "having no more interest in life," then it's time to give them a ginseng supplement to bring back to them their vitality, fitness, and zest for life.

Problems of menopause such as bouts of depression, headaches, mental weakness, tension, and sleeplessness are clearly improved as well. (See also chapter 14.) Several clinical studies are still under way to show that ginseng can lower blood fat and blood pressure, whereas its lowering of the blood sugar is already an established fact. There can be no doubt that the next goals of scientific investigation will be to prove positive effects on the immune system.

In our view, the "chronic fatigue syndrome" recently experienced by so many people in the United States can be cured in less than three months with the help of a good, highly concentrated, standardized ginseng extract, possibly in combination with vitamins, minerals, and trace elements. For it is truly no secret that physical and mental fatigue are linked to stress combined with vitamin and mineral deficiency due to an unnatural life style and a poor diet. The human body consists of about 60 billion cells, in which metabolic processes are continually occuring. Vitamins, minerals, and trace elements play a decisive role in all of them; for example, they are important for the formation of bone and blood and for the protection of the cells. If we don't supply our body with a sufficient quantity of these life essentials, we cannot expect our cells to give their best, and the inevitable result will be malfunction and terrible fatigue. Therefore, people who know that their diet is inadequate should take the opportunity and use such a combined ginseng product as a main supplement.

OUR PERSONAL EXPERIENCE

We personally made a few experiments with ginseng preparations when we went on long and difficult mountaineering tours. Not only we and our two elder children but also a friend of ours, a very experienced mountain guide, have discovered the great help that a mouthful of ginseng tonic or one or two chewable ginseng tabs can provide when we feel really at the end of our strength. Because we are not very well-trained hikers but love the mountains and love adventures that challenge us physically, we never go on a hike without a bottle of ginseng extract in our backpack. So far, it has given us new strength and endurance every time we truly needed it.

~ 17 ~

HERBS FOR PLEASURE

If there were no plants we would not be here. We breathe in what they breathe out. That is how we learn from them.

Keetoowah, Cherokee healer

Besides being aware of the medicinal uses of herbs, we should never forget that they are also available in abundance for the preparation of pleasantly flavored and refreshing herbal teas and for making our foods more interesting and delicious. Thus, not only are herbs appropriate when a particular medicinal effect is sought, they are perfect when you are feeling on top of the world as well.

There is great pleasure to be had from handling and experimenting with herbs, for they are one of nature's greatest gifts; they gently stimulate all our senses with their perfumes, colors, and flavors. In contrast to herbal teas, coffee and common "black" tea, the familiar hot drinks, cause damage to your nerves and put a great strain on the stomach. Have you also discovered that their stimulating effect weakens as your intake increases? Among our friends and associates, anyone who has tried our herbal teas over a period of time has gradually changed over from habitual coffee drinking to the enjoyment of herbal teas instead.

Every health-conscious family is also concerned about healthy beverages. Pure water is wonderful but not always satisfying. Commercially manufactured drinks such as colas and soda pops contain large quantities of sugar or artificial sweeteners, and the continuous consumption of even so-called natural sodas will irritate the stomach because of the carbonic acid they contain. Often, as we have observed, such drinks "pervert" the flavor preferences of children. Fruit juices are frequently much too concentrated to be enjoyed with meals, and alcoholic beverages—if consumed at all—should be reserved for special occasions. So herbal teas offer an ideal solution for the whole family. Available in an almost infinite variety of flavors, they can be enjoyed hot or cold depending upon your preference and the time of year. (An interesting side note: cool drinks in winter and warm drinks in summer are quite "natural." For example, next time you are seeking refreshment on a hot summer day, try a cup of warm herbal tea and experience for yourself how long its thirst-quenching benefits last.) Herbal tea blends can be mixed to provide the perfect compliment for every meal. And because herbal tea is like pure water in that it contains no calories but simply vitamins and minerals, it's the ideal choice for those members of the family who have to watch their weight.

Many of our friends compose their own personal blends of herbal teas, just as we do. During the year, they collect from their gardens and the surrounding countryside the various herbs, flowers, leaves, and fruits as they unfold and ripen. This starts in the spring with cowslips, violets, birch leaves, elder flowers, strawberry leaves, and linden blossoms. In summer come the herbs such as rose blossoms, dandelion, calendula, balm, peppermint, and sage leaves, blackberry shoots, horsetail, stinging nettle, St. Johnswort, mullein, mallow, lavender, chamomile blossoms, rosemary and plaintain leaves, thyme, yarrow, small flowered willow-herb, and goldenrod. Last of all, in late autumn the rose hips are gathered. As the harvesting continues everything is laid out on large cloths or wrapping paper, up in the attic where it's warm and perfect for drying, and by the season's end the household boasts a wonderful assortment of colorful herbs.

If you choose to carry out a similar family herbal tea project, be sure to encourage the children to join in. Children from the age of one year up love to handle herbs, to discover their different qualities, colors, shapes, and fragrances, and to help with plucking, chopping, and packaging the herbs. This makes your own herbal mixtures naturally very special. At Christmas time, you can package your home tea mixtures as unique gifts or even give scented herbal pillows or sachets to family and friends. Take care to use up your supply of herbs before next spring, when nature will provide you with fresh new herbs to enjoy.

The beautifully balanced tea mixture below, which we created when we first became engaged with herbs, we simply call "Household Tea." We still enjoy it even after all these years. It is particularly suitable for drinking with the evening meal or as a nightcap before retiring.

🜚 Household Tea 🜚

7 parts balm leaves
4 parts cocoa pod
3 parts peppermint leaves
3 parts hibiscus flowers
1 part chamomile flowers
1 part cinnamon bark
½ part calendula flowers
½ part cornflower blooms

Our Refresher Tea, by contrast, is a suitable breakfast tea, though naturally you can enjoy it anytime during the day as well. The addition of maté makes this blend an excellent morning beverage and activity tea. Since maté contains caffeine (but much less than coffee or black tea), those who wish to do so can substitute 5 parts rosemary leaves for maté in the following formula. (We haven't noticed any significant difference between the two mixtures.)

🜚 Refresher Tea 🜚

5 parts maté leaves
5 parts whole rose hips
4 parts hibiscus flowers
3 parts raspberry leaves
3 parts blackberry leaves

As we have mentioned several times, we attach great importance to guiding the taste preferences of children in a different direction than is normally the case today. Just as in many parts of America young children are given soda pop and cola regularly, it is usual in Europe to ply the baby right from the start with tea sweetened with sugar. This fact was the cause of a great scandal in Germany some years ago when it

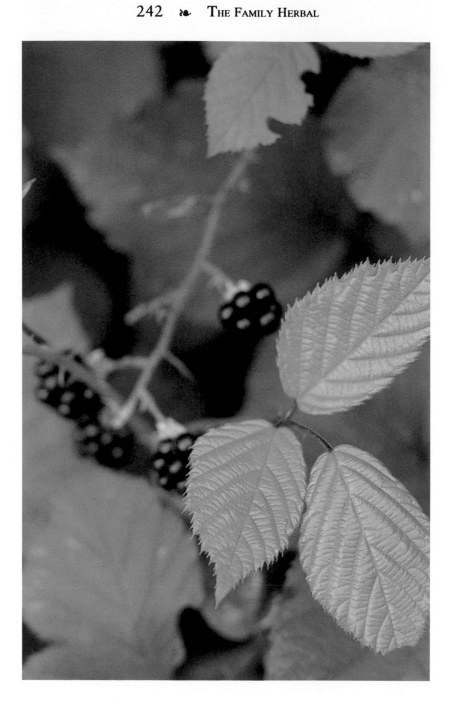

BLACKBERRY LEAVES   *Rubus fruticosus*

was discovered that habitual sucking of bottles filled with instant sugar-based tea led to tooth damage of catastrophic proportions. At the time there was scarcely any mention of the long-term effects beyond the ruination of the baby's milk teeth, but such teas, which consist of up to 60 percent sugar, inevitably condition an infant's taste preference toward sweet things, a conditioning that is likely to remain for life. For these reasons, babies should be given only sugar-free teas to quench their thirst. The following blend of herbal tea also contains so-called carminatives (antiflatulence herbs), as is usual in herbal teas designed for children and babies. It is therefore suitable for children of all ages, even infants.

⚬ Children's Tea ⚬

4 parts fennel seeds
4 parts rose hips
3 parts hibiscus flowers
3 parts balm leaves
3 parts cowslip flowers
1 part caraway seed
¾ part peppermint leaves
½ part chamomile

Even those parents who prefer instant herbal teas now have a better solution. As mentioned on page 36, a water-soluble protein base has been developed that makes it possible to manufacture high-quality, sugar-free, instant herbal teas.

As you can see from the recipes given in this chapter, a certain range of herbs is particularly suitable for the preparation of "beverage" herbal teas. These are primarily the following: balm leaves, hibiscus flowers, St. Johnswort, elder flowers, linden blossoms, strawberry leaves, raspberry leaves, blackberry leaves, rose hips, orange blossoms, cocoa pods, cinnamon bark, and cowslip flowers. Vervain and yellow bedstraw are included to produce particularly pleasing aromas. All of these herbs can be freely mixed with each other. It is impossible for you to go wrong.

BLACKBERRY AND RASPBERRY LEAVES

The leaves of the blackberry (*Rubus fruticosus*), which grows luxuriantly in neglected gardens, by fences, palisades, field drains, and at the edge of woods, provide us with a marvelous basis for herbal tea mixtures of all types. The blackberry plant's unmistakable characteristics include its jagged-edged leaves and its shoots, which are often yards long and frequently form impenetrable thickets thanks to their numerous sharp thorns. The blackberry does not bloom at any particular time. It carries blossom, ripe fruit, and unripe fruit all at the same time. The harvest is made in the spring and early summer, long before the berries ripen, and consists of gathering only the tender young shoots and the light green leaves. When dried and extracted in hot water, the leaves have a fine flavor that is reminiscent of fine Indian or Chinese teas. In earlier times, when such Asian teas were unaffordably expensive, blackberry leaves were treated by the same fermentation process as that used for black tea and served as a substitute for the latter. The surrogate "black" tea hardly differs in appearance from the "real" tea, yet is much healthier since it contains no caffeine. Blackberry leaves alone produce a perfectly pleasant breakfast tea, possibly with the addition of a little lemon. They should always be employed when it is necessary to subdue or harmonize a dominant component in an herbal tea blend, such as a bitter taste. Finally, blackberry leaves are not without medicinal effect. The large quantities of tannic acid they contain provide their astringent (drawing-together) property and help to "brake" diarrhea. Raspberry leaves are employed in exactly the same manner.

STRAWBERRY LEAVES

Wild strawberries, or wood strawberries (*Fragaria vesca*), are beloved not only because of their delicious fruit; they too provide tender green leaves in the spring that make a pleasant-tasting household tea. One of the ways this low-growing perennial multiplies is to send out runners that grow along the surface of the ground, sending down new roots into the soil. The tiny white flowers develop into fleshy berries that are valued in folk medicine for the treatment of a whole variety of disorders. A herbal tea prepared from the leaves is also mildly astringent and is effective against diarrhea. Strawberry leaves, like blackberry and raspberry leaves, are ideal, flavorsome additions to any "nonspecific" household herb tea.

THIRST QUENCHERS

When it is desirable to impart a fresh acidic flavor to a herbal tea, then

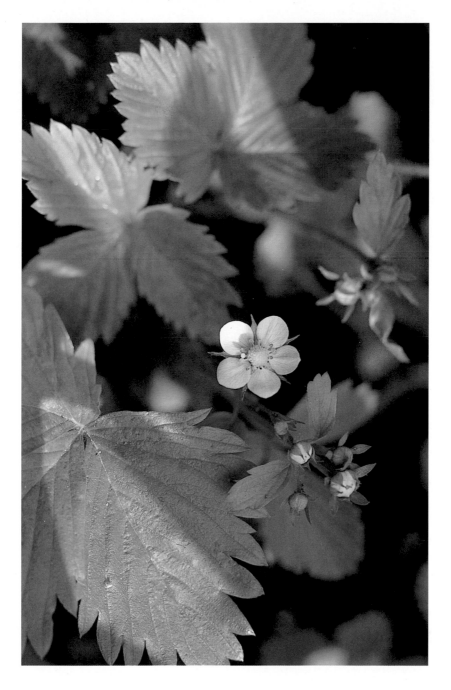

STRAWBERRY LEAVES *Fragaria vesica*

the herbs of choice are hibiscus flowers and rose hips. Pure hibiscus tea is deep red in color and has a very refreshing flavor. Whether drunk hot or ice cold, it is a very good thirst quencher during the hot season. Whenever we go walking or hill climbing we take along a thermos of tea prepared from hibiscus flowers, rose hips, and balm leaves. Flavored with a little lemon juice and perhaps a bit of honey, this is a wonderful drink for nipping thirst in the bud. It is also just right for active sportsmen and sportswomen.

Rose Hips

Hips are the accessory fruit of the common wild rose (*Rosa canina*), also known as the dog rose. The deep red fruits decorate old rose bushes in autumn even after the leaves and flowers are gone. If you remove the thin layer of fruity flesh, you will find inside densely packed, hard, and remarkably hairy little seeds. Hips can be either dried whole or cut up with the seeds removed. In any case, they become very hard and need an extraction time of fifteen to twenty minutes or boiling for five to ten minutes. In order to prepare a hip conserve, the seeds must ultimately be removed—a very laborious task! Such a conserve is very rich in vitamin C, a characteristic that applies to hip tea as well. For this reason, hips are often included in herbal teas intended for the treatment of colds and chills and are rightly employed for prevention of these conditions. We include hips in many tea blends because of their fine, acidic flavor.

Favorite Winter Beverages

Every year at Christmas, we make up a little gift for the customers in our pharmacy. Some years ago we composed a fruit tea blend with a particularly aromatic flavor, one that has since become a great favorite in our household and around town. Its name translates as Festivity Tea. It is a real winter tea warmer, a tea whose flavor is reminiscent of Christmas cookies and mulled wine. (We find it perfect for long winter evenings when we linger in front of the fireplace.) The recipe is as follows:

ᴥ Festivity Tea ᴥ

4 parts apple pieces
3 parts rose hips without seeds
3 parts balm leaves

3 parts hibiscus flowers
2 parts cocoa pod
2 parts cinnamon bark
1 part orange blossom
1 part orange peel
½ part lemon peel
½ part crushed cloves

The recipe also serves as a base for a nonalcoholic punch to be made at Christmas or on New Year's Eve. For this purpose various fruit juices and spices are added to the Festivity Tea; the resulting savory mixture has delighted our guests (including children) on many occasions. The amazing thing is that this beverage tastes just like a genuine punch although it does not contain any alcohol.

🎔 Nonalcoholic Festivity Punch 🎔

1 quart Festivity Tea
¾ quart black currant juice
¾ quart red grape juice
juice of 3 oranges
juice of 1 lemon
grated peel of 1 unsprayed orange
whole peel of 1 unsprayed orange
3 cinnamon sticks, broken into pieces
20 whole cloves
⅛ teaspoon ground nutmeg
⅛ teaspoon ground star anise
⅛ teaspoon allspice
3 tablespoons of concentrated apple juice

Place all of the liquid ingredients in a large pot and add the spices. Bring the mixture to a boil, then reduce heat and simmer for about fifteen minutes. Strain through a sieve before serving.

SUMMER BEVERAGES

There are also many natural opportunities in summer to produce delicious things with herbs. At all our festivities we take care to provide something special for the children as well as for those who have no taste for alcoholic beverages. That's how our Sage Punch was created, a drink

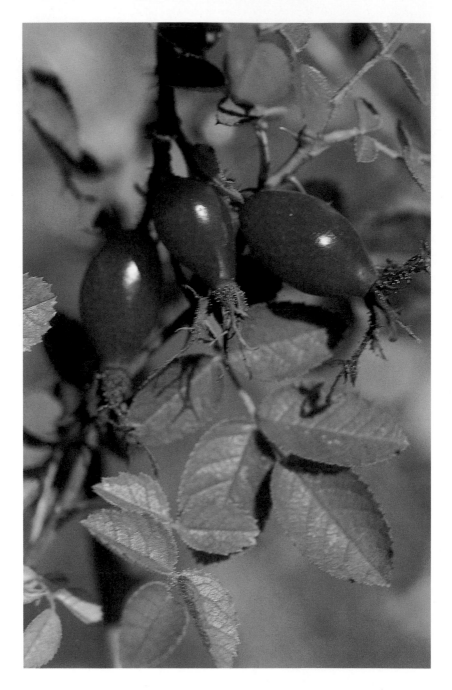

ROSE HIPS   *Rosa canina*

that tastes fantastic and is also very agreeable. Here's the recipe:

❧ Sage Punch ☙

2 to 3 quarts sage tea (made from 2 handfuls freshly
  gathered sage leaves)
2 cans mandarin orange segments (without juice)
2 to 3 tablespoonsful honey
1 bottle of nonalcoholic champagne
  (or regular champagne if desired)

Brew the sage tea several hours in advance, stir in the honey, and cool in the refrigerator until chilled. Then add the fruit, and top off with champagne. Serve chilled, decorated with fresh sage leaves.

Another recipe is the favorite summer drink of our family. We call it simply Summer Tea.

❧ Summer Tea ☙

1 quart tea made from equal parts of fresh peppermint
  and balm leaves as well as dried hibiscus flowers
1 large shot of elder flower syrup (see below) or
  maple syrup
Juice of 1 lemon

Brew the tea and allow it to cool, add the syrup and lemon juice and serve chilled over ice.

Elder flower syrup is a real specialty that may be used to flavor any herb tea. It is produced from fresh elder flowers and has a fine and very fragrant aroma. It can also be used to flavor sweet dishes such as ice creams or fruit salads.

❧ Elder Flower Syrup ☙

50 clusters of elder flowers
3 quarts water
1½ kg. (3⅓ lb.) granulated maple sugar or
  granulated sugar cane juice

Lay the freshly harvested elder flowers in the water in a large pot and allow to stand for twenty-four hours. (This makes the water very aromatic.) Strain off the flowers through a sieve covered with cheesecloth so that no plant residues remain in the water, not even minute particles.

Combine the water and sweetener in the pot and boil it for five minutes. Immediately pour into large clean jars or bottles and seal. The syrup can be kept for one year as long as it is stored in the refrigerator after being opened. Our attempts to use honey as an alternate sweetener in this recipe have only resulted in failure. First, the blossom aroma becomes almost completely masked by that of the honey, and second, the honey-based syrup will not keep. This recipe traditionally called for white sugar, but since we try to avoid white sugar as much as possible, we replace it with granulated maple sugar or granulated sugar cane juice.

Elder flowers have many uses in the spring. The traditional elder cakes, for example, are simply clusters of elder flowers dipped in pancake batter and then deep-fried. Another traditional European peasant recipe has been used for hundreds of years to produce elder must (must is an old-fashioned, naturally carbonated, sodalike drink). In our family we make a marvelous Elder Pop, a very refreshing and vitalizing drink. Although it does require a little practice to master its preparation and preservation, it's worth trying if you can find fresh elder flowers.

⟡ Elder Pop ⟡

10 quarts water
30 to 50 clusters elder flowers
1 kg. (2 lb.) maple sugar or granulated sugar cane juice
3 unsprayed lemons, sliced
Juice of 1 lemon

Place the water, flowers, and lemon slices in a large stoneware pot or crock and allow to stand for twenty-four hours. Then strain off the flowers and add the lemon juice and the sweetener. Stir well and allow the mixture to stand for another twenty-four hours. A slight fermentation process will take place, and the pop is then ready to drink. It has a refreshing flavor and is an excellent thirst quencher. The pop may also be poured into bottles, carefully corked, and allowed to stand in a cool cellar. After three to four weeks a quantity of carbonic acid will have been produced and the pop will prickle like champagne when drunk cold or chilled.

Peppermint Cocktails

Of course one of the most refreshing iced herbal teas is that made from fresh peppermint leaves. According to taste you can drink it plain or with a squirt of lemon juice. You can also try it with a bit of maple syrup or concentrated apple or pear juice. Moreover, such herbal iced drinks can be easily garnished to look every bit as appetizing as the most exotic cocktail. One of our favorites, which we've dubbed the Mint Iceberg, makes the perfect climax to a festive summer meal. One or two scoops of lemon sorbet are placed in a chilled champagne glass, which is then filled with ice cold peppermint tea. Don't forget to add a fresh sprig of peppermint leaf as decoration. Similarly, a slice of fruit slipped over the edge of a glass or a few floating rose petals will make any herbal drink more attractive and pleasurable. Peppermint can also be used to create a light summer sorbet.

❧ Peppermint Sorbet ☙

6 oz. granulated sugar cane juice
1 quart water
2 oz. fresh mint leaves
½ oz. dried peppermint leaves
juice of ½ lemon

Put the sweetener and water in a saucepan and bring to a boil for one minute. Infuse the dried and fresh leaves in the syrup and allow to cool. Finally, drain and squeeze out the mint leaves. Add the lemon juice (more or less according to taste), and place the liquid in an ice cream maker. After about thirty minutes a very light and refreshing sorbet will be ready. Decorate with fresh mint leaves and serve immediately!

CULINARY HERBS

Recipes abound for delightful hors d'oeuvres, main courses, side dishes, soups, salads, and desserts whose preparation involves herbs. More than any other cuisine, Italian cooking incorporates herbs in almost every dish. This is one reason why we love Italian food so much. Just thinking about such classical dishes as spaghetti with fresh sage or garlic, chicken with rosemary, and saffron risotto makes our mouths water with anticipation. Then again, even a simple meal featuring roasted potatoes with thyme or a light sorrel soup is a joy for both the palate and the body. But here we had better stop, for a treatise on the herbal refinements of cooking would require a whole book in itself. Instead, we would like to end with a chapter of ideas for creating your own herb garden.

❧ 18 ❧

CREATE YOUR OWN HERB GARDEN

The foolish run
The clever wait
The wise go in the garden
> Rabindranath Tagore

This last chapter comes back to where we began, with the question, How can I best learn about herbs? We invite you now to create your own herb garden even if you have only a very small area available; a square of 15 x 15 feet (5 x 5 meters) would be sufficient for a start. The herbs incorporated in our model garden are predominantly the same as those described in the various chapters of this book. For more detailed information on their botanical data, their healing power, and the ways of using them, please look up the respective chapters and pictures.

HISTORICAL EXAMPLES AND DEMANDS OF TODAY

In dealing with the subject of herb gardens, we can be considerably helped by studying the great classical examples in Europe. The most beautiful ones today can still be found in Great Britain, that amazing paradise of gardening fanatics. France, Belgium, and Holland also offer several splendid examples that need to be seen. Without exception, those old exquisite herb gardens were conceived as a special section in a huge park surrounding an old homestead, the country house of a noble family, a palace, or a castle. Nowadays some of these residences have been transformed into splendid hotels, and consequently their extended gardens are still well kept, including the kitchen gardens, once again operated for the refinement of the restaurant's cuisine.

The other historical model, exclusively oriented toward the healing benefits of herbs, are and have always been the herb gardens belonging to ancient cloisters and monasteries. In the Middle Ages and the following centuries, these botanical treasures have been maintained as an important and reputable source of high-quality medications throughout Europe.

A mixture of both the culinary and the medicinal aspects can be found in the simpler rural form or the old-fashioned peasant's herb garden. This type, in our opinion, comes closest to the desires of today's gardeners, since it perfectly integrates the three major claims of a modern herb garden: to be *beautiful and decorative* in supplying both fresh and dried plants; to be *practical,* so that we can make good use of our herbs for the natural healthcare of our family; and to be *delicious,* providing us with seasoning subtleties for cooking that we cannot buy. Surely a few herbs will also be used as vegetables, and of course, there is no reason why you should not complement your vegetable garden with seasoning herbs or plant your herb garden with a selection of vegetables. Some of the herbs are worth being cultivated just for the sake of their scent, both fresh and dried, and the love of their natural aromas is one more good reason to create your own herb garden. Potpourris are another charming invention of English garden lovers handed down to us as a lovely tradition, and together with aromatherapy, the use of potpourris has become fashionable again these days. Also, we observe in garden and home journals as well as in books that the most competent culinary professionals fall back more and more on herbs for table and plate decorations.

As mentioned in chapters 2 and 3, we started our career as herbalists by dealing with wild herbs. However, since we have our own garden in which more than 150 herbs grow, we find it very handy to have them so close at our disposal at all times. Whether for demonstrating an herb at a lecture, blending a delicious early-morning tea, treating a skin rash, eliminating a wart, or seasoning our salads, we would not want to be without our own garden herbs.

An Old-Fashioned Symmetrical Layout

There is no reason why in a garden, like ours, herbs could not grow anywhere, according to their own needs, and be completely mixed among the other flowers, bushes, trees, and groundcovers. However, we find that the symmetrical pattern of the old-fashioned herb or kitchen garden has a very special charm. Nowhere else will you find scents and aromas so subtle, shades and color nuances so delicate, shapes and structures so attractive. Some herb gardeners are especially proud of growing their herbs in as many species variations as possible. This is certainly a fascinating task; however, it is limited by space.

We have tried to capture the special attraction of the old ornamental style in a mandala-like pattern with a clearly marked center point.

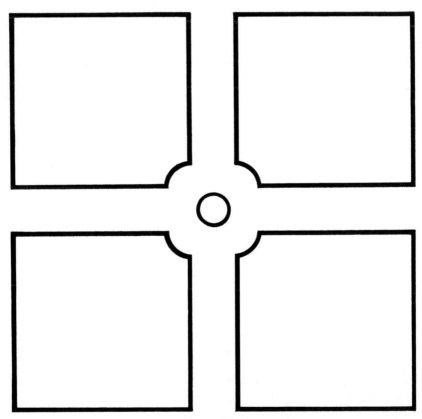

FIGURE 12
Herb Garden Design

As a tribute to tradition, we suggest that you surround the four beds by low box hedges and divide them by four paved pathways. The center point could be marked, depending upon the size of the whole garden or section, by an arbor veiled with roses, a small water fountain, a column bearing a statue or piece of art, a trimmed tree, or just a bright colorful plant in a big pot. If you decide for the latter, we suggest a round shaped orange or lime tree (if climate conditions allow) or a large ball-shaped laurel berry (which must be put inside during cold winters). Also, a large standard daisy in a pretty pot can look very attractive.

DIFFERENT WAYS OF GROUPING

The seasoning and healing plants that we suggest for the four beds are grouped according to their characters and colors, and they are arranged in such a way as to orient everything toward the center. This means that the tallest plants—trees and high bushes—are positioned in the far corners, and the other plants diminish in size toward the center and the pathways.

In reflecting on the possible choices for the composition of the various plants, one could of course choose numerous other principles. You could arrange the herbs according to their natural habitat, which would certainly make much sense, e.g., the moisture-loving plants from the swamplands in one corner, those that love the sun and can bear dry soil in another corner, those that need shade under the protection of trees and bushes, and so forth. However, it seems to us that this would demand a lot of space, which often is not available, and extensive preconditioning of the soil, which often is too costly. Several herb gardens recently laid out in Germany group the plants according to their medicinal indications: for example, one bed of herbs useful for indigestion, another of herbs good for the nervous system, another of herbs that heal the organs of the respiratory tract, etc. This principle is excellent for demonstration and teaching purposes. One could even group plants according to their astrological relationships with planets or signs of the zodiac. There are really many choices.

Our composition is guided by both practical and esthetic aspects. It is important that the gardener be able to easily reach those herbs that are often cut and regrow fast, whereas the ones that are harvested only once a year are placed further in the back. Of course, we cannot guarantee that all the suggested herbs will grow in one and the same bed. This is before all else a question of the soil and climate conditions, and it is a good idea to arm oneself with patience in order to find out where each herb loves to be and perhaps to change their positions in the course of a few years.

PLANT RELATIONSHIPS

Nevertheless, we have considered, as much as possible, plant friendships and enmities that are either known among gardeners or part of our personal experience. For it is a fact that among plants, too, there are tendencies of sympathy and antipathy, and it is extremely interesting to observe them. The most memorable experience of such observations has been the "behavior" of a hop plant in our herb garden. Right next to it, at a distance of about 4 feet (1.20 meters), there grew a tall plant of valerian, a mugwort, and an angelica. As soon as the first hop scion came out of the earth, it tried to climb up one of the valerian stems. When I (Barbara) took it and directed it toward the mugwort, it turned away, showing a definite aversion for this partner. When I wound the scion around the angelica leaves, the hop showed the same reaction and withdrew. With speed, it returned back to the valerian and continued twining up this neighbor. Repeated corrections through my interference had the same result again and again: valerian and hop seemed to love each other. When I realized that often these same herbs are combined in tea blends for sleeplessness, my newest interest and hobby was born: the observation of botanical friendships or partnerships in relation to their combination in medicinal tea blends and other herbal preparations.

PLANTS FOR YOUR HERB GARDEN SQUARE

Bed One
Bed one contains a big tall bush of wild roses, placed here not for the sake of the flowers or petals but for the fruits, the rosehips, which will decorate their corner with red patches throught fall and winter and possibly even be used in your Christmas garlands. Two blackberry bushes provide their fruits in late summer and are a source of fresh leaves to enrich your house tea all through the year. Comfrey root can be dug, dried, and powdered for poultices, and its rather large and tall bush

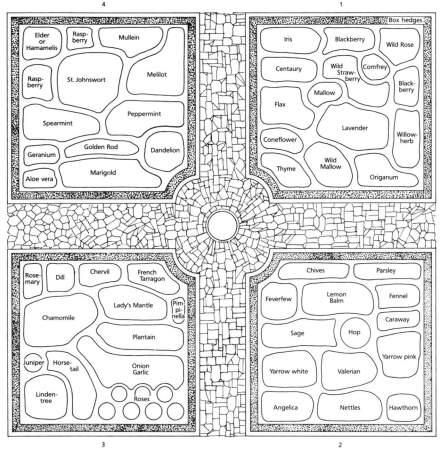

FIGURE 13

Plants for Each Section of the Herb Garden

provides shade for the wood strawberries, whose leaves can also be added to any unspecific tea blend. Irises in the left corner will please with their beauty and elegance and also provide their roots (only after several years!) for various uses. Centaury is probably difficult to find in a nursery; it is a very pretty pink flower whose bitterness is absolutely amazing. Cone-flower should be there, mainly for demonstration, decoration, and learning, because the whole plant extract of *Echinacea purpurea* or *pallida,* well known as an effective immune booster, cannot be prepared easily. Mallow flowers and ripening fruits are most effective when freshly picked and added to a tea against bronchitis or sore throat (use only warm, not boiling water for extraction).

For their beauty's sake, we have also incorporated a patch of garden mallow, available in beautiful shades from bright white and pale pink to darkest purple. The flowers of these tall varieties can also be dried and used for tea. Although they are not important medicinally, since they do not contain as many mucins as the wild mallow, they add a lovely sour taste to any tea blend and are very decorative for potpourris as well. Willow-herb is a real weed in the sense that it grows on every soil, but mind its spreading seeds in late summer—if you do not control it, it will take over the entire space in two seasons! The low-growing or creeping thyme (there are numerous variations) is excellent when used fresh in soups and stews, or on lamb chops and pizza. It can easily be dried for the winter. Origanum is its spicy companion, best loved in Italian food and never omitted from a hearty spaghetti sauce. Lavender flowers are a wonderful addition to a refreshing bath as well as a major ingredient of potpourris for the bathroom. Flax brings forth the most lovely, tender, small sky-blue flowers. Although you could harvest the linseeds from this plant, we do not encourage you to do so because the work is too tedious. But if you have a piece of clothing made out of true linen, you can verify its origin by comparing its fibers with the fine fibers packed inside the flax stems and realize what a useful plant this is.

Bed Two

In bed two the hawthorn bush is the tallest plant, providing white blossoms in spring, green leaves in summer, and red berries in fall for all those who need support for their heart. From all three parts, a pleasant heart tea can be prepared. With the hawthorn berries, you will also be sure to attract many birds. Angelica can grow as tall as a man and bears decorative umbrella-like flowers. It is one of those empowering bitter-aromatic roots that help digestion and provide "yang" energy. The stinging nettles and, if you wish, other more decorative species of nettles, are given a space in the back so they will not burn your legs when you walk by. Even though they do not seem to be very friendly fellows, you should use them abundantly in your blood-cleansing teas against allergies and all poisons you will to eliminate from your system. It is advisable to pick the leaves with gloves on when you harvest them, either for a fresh vegetable dish in spring or for your flushing teas and mixtures. Once they have taken root, you do not need to be afraid: Even if you cut them off completely, they will regrow without fail.

Valerian is again an herb that is rather difficult to harvest and pre-pare because the root must be dug, dried, and cut or professionally extracted. Unlike the root, the blossoms have a very pleasant odor, and the entire living plant is one of those excellent companions for vegetable plants that help their neighbors grow better and keep unwanted insects away. As described earlier in this chapter, there is a real love story going on between hop and valerian. For the hop plant, it is necessary to erect a rather tall frame, pole, or vertical wire. Otherwise, it cannot climb upward as it should. You certainly won't harvest enough hop to brew your own beer, but you could gather the hop cones in September or October and add them to your sleeping tea or fill them into a sleeping pillow as a very effective aromatherapy against sleeplessness. By the way, a hop shoot harvested in its entirety in fall is very decorative when hung on the ceiling or wall or around an entrance like a garland. It dries beau-tifully without changing much of its shape or color. When it comes to yarrow, you should definitely try to get at least the regular white one and the slightly bigger pink one and let them grow into big patches, because of their decorative value. It has been observed that some species of the yarrow family do not grow well together. That is why, as a pre-caution, we have separated them into two groups and planted the me-diator valerian between them. The flower-bearing stalks of yarrow can easily be dried in fall and worked into dry bunches. For medicinal pur-poses, the entire herb can be prepared as a tea or bath for menstrual cramps and digestive problems.

Fennel and caraway are two good friends whose seeds not only make an effective tea against bloating but also are best suited for seasoning home-made breads and potato dishes. Then comes sage with its numer-ous variations. Be sure to have the regular garden sage among them, and use the strong-smelling leaves fresh for Italian pasta dishes, and in winter—dried or fresh—as a gargle for sore throat. With balm also, it is easy to find more than one species. Balm isn't particular at all, thriving luxuriantly in big cushions so that you can harvest large quantities of the green herb and prepare nerve-calming baths and teas at any time. Remember that the aroma is best when the herb is harvested before flow-ering time, but if you leave part of the plant, the blossoms will attract bees and butterflies in masses. Chives and parsley need to be present in abundance in a good herb garden, and throughout spring, summer, and fall, you should never prepare a full meal without these health-bringing herbs. By the way, you surely will use much less salt if you use herbs for achieving spicy and piquant tastes. Feverfew bears lovely white flowers with a yellow dot in the center, and its characteristic leaves and typical scent give evidence of its belonging to the chrysanthemum family. For people with chronic migraines, feverfew is a must. It might even be your savior if you eat one fresh leaf every day.

Bed Three

In bed three we have placed a linden tree, which you will adore just as we do because of the heavenly sweet scent of its flowers when they are in full bloom in early summer. If you can afford the space, allow a little open area around it so that you can sit underneath it, either on grass or on a bench, and enjoy its strong healing vibration. You should not fail to collect a bag full of the blossoms to make a tea or footbath for nipping a cold in the bud by inducing perspiration and assisting your immune defense. Underneath the linden tree, you can try to plant horsetail, but this is a rather peculiar fellow who needs very special soil conditions. Its natural friend and neighbor in the wild heathland, juniper, should get along well with horsetail and help it to take root. Juniper is a narrow, vertically growing bush, whose berries are a strong diuretic agent—much like horsetail—but must be dosed very carefully because of possible side effects. A few whole juniper berries steamed with sauerkraut or added to a hearty mixed vegetable soup add a very interesting touch.

Along one of the sides of the bed you can plant as many pretty, strong-scented roses as you like. We would prefer so-called old roses, either taller standard plants or creeping and hanging species. Since there will be no more other strong colors in this bed, you can pick any shade. Here, the roses are mainly valued for their petals and scent, and you may use them for decoration in all possible ways, dried or fresh. One of the newer creations has been to let loose fresh rose petals float in a flat bowl of water or to hang dried ones threaded on long strings or thin wires on chandeliers. In the south of France, it has long been customary to plant roses in the vicinity of onions and garlic in order to enhance the roses' smell. Little known is the fact that onions, leeks, and garlic look very pretty with their flower-balls in white, gray, and violet-blue when they are allowed to bloom. Besides their extremely healthful bulbs, they also offer their stems, which can season your salads when cut into small rings. A very delicate and rare but most intense cleanser among these plants is the wild garlic, which appears for only a few weeks in spring with its juicy green leaves and tender white blossoms. If you are lucky enough to find it and make it at home in your garden, benefit from it for your spring cleansing cure and eat all of its parts raw as a rare delicacy.

Plantain may be difficult to find in a nursery. If you are eager to grow it, you can transplant it from meadows and grass walks. In any case, its leaves are the best cough remedy we have, often used for the preparation of a cough syrup or cough tea, and are effective in the immediate care of stinging nettle "burns"! Lady's mantle is indispensable for florists, who enjoy binding big round flower bunches in summer because the nicely shaped leaves and yellow-green filigreed flowers are perfect fillers for every bouquet. Women who have problems with menstruation or menopause will appreciate the help of this unpretentious herb. Another important herb for women is chamomile, whose flowers, fresh or dried, are a great remedy for skin problems, wounds, sinus inflammations, and a host of other complaints; chamomile can be used in the form of tea, extract, bath, or inhalation. As an attractive variation, Roman chamomile which has larger, filled blossoms, could be incorporated into your garden if the climate is warm enough. Dill, chervil, French tarragon, and pimpinella are all greens that refine, with their delicate aromas, raw salads, dips, dressings, and white cheese as well as exquisite sauces, vegetable dishes, and soups. For persons with poor blood circulation, rosemary leaves are the natural remedy as tea or bath. Gourmets often prefer a roast of lamb, venison, or other red meat cooked with sprigs of rosemary.

Bed Four

The tallest and most dominant bush in the fourth bed is either elder or *Hamamelis*. We personally like elder because it is a very traditional and distinctive plant, well adapted to colder climates. Its blossoms can be harvested in spring for the preparation of elder pop, the outstandingly aromatic flower syrup, or various tea blends against colds and flus. Also, the black berries that the bush presents in fall are very healthful and rich in minerals. The problem with elder, however, is that it does not tolerate other plants in its vicinity; it truly is a "killer" plant very similar to the birch tree, which equally demands a huge area around itself as its exclusive territory. That is why, if space is limited, we hesitate to recommend an elder plant, whereas with witch hazel (*Hamamelis virginiana*) we are sure you will be happy because this bush will amaze you with its strangely formed yellow blossoms in the middle of winter. The leaves and bark can be used for the treatment of inflammations in the mouth and throat, and there are numerous cosmetic creams for natural skin care as well as medicinal preparations for the treatment of varicose veins, wounds, and diarrhea containing *Hamamelis* extracts. Two raspberry bushes are its neighbors, offering to us delicious berries in summer and young shoots and leaves for tea all year long.

Mullein flowers tend to become very tall and stalky in late summer as they grow out of their silvery velvet rosette on the ground. As the blossoms slowly open upward along the torch, they can be harvested and dried for an effective bronchitis tea. This plant is a biennial, developing only the rosette in the first year and the flowering stalks in the second year. St. Johnswort, with its yellow glowing flowers, brings in the climax of summer and enriches us with a tasty tea for nervous disorders and depressions. Melilot, or yellow clover, is known for its lovely fragrance and calming properties. Harvested in full bloom and dried, it makes an important ingredient of a sleeping pillow. This little comforter may be a good solution for your overworked husband or crying baby.

Of course, we can't leave out the large family of the peppermints. Since peppermint and spearmint with all their hybrids are much loved during the hot season as thirst-quenching iced teas, we also want to grow lots of them. The homemade peppermint sorbet or the cocktail decorated with the top-leaves of the plant can surely become a highlight at your summer party, and gallstone patients will find that warm peppermint tea helps the gallbladder to calm down and release the tension. The leaves of aloe vera—if your climate allows its growth—can be used as a first-aid treatment for burns, including sunburns, if sliced open and placed on the burn.

Dandelion is another one of those tenacious weeds that are not generally provided in garden centers but grow abundantly in meadows. Its leaves taste deliciously bitter and are great medications for the liver, gallbladder, stomach, and kidneys. Dandelion is a must for all who want to cleanse the body and flush it out. In France and in Germany, two varieties are now offered in shops as salad greens. Goldenrod, another pretty yellow-blossomed herb, flushes the kidneys and bladder when made into a tea. Last but not least, the curved seeds of pot marigold (calendula) must be sown in spring, and you will observe how this flower spreads itself during the next few years, although it is an annual plant. Since there are filled and unfilled blossoms as well as orange and yellow ones, it is worth trying to get as many varieties as possible. Marigold will bloom all through the summer and fall and adorn your herb garden with its intense glow. Besides putting the flowers in vases and using them in rustic arrangements, be sure to collect and dry the flower petals and add them to your house blend or your potpourris. The scented geranium has been chosen for the garden because, by its intense odor, it keeps away parasites.

TENDING YOUR HERB GARDEN

In the maintenance of the herb garden, the major mistake we have seen over and over again is too much fertilizing. Bear in mind that in most cases, herbs by their nature of being weeds thrive in very poor soils. Giving them lots of organic fertilizer (chemical ones should not even be considered!) causes them to grow "out of their size," making them look weak and disorderly. Except for the scented roses, it is a fact that in an herb garden you can hardly fertilize too little.

It goes without saying that in an organic herb garden, herbicides and pesticides have no place whatsoever. You wouldn't be so naive as to expect healing or beneficial effects from plants that you had first poisoned by chemicals! And of course you must stick to this principle even if bugs or snails eat your plants and harvest. Rather than killing the bugs, you should go about carefully establishing a healthy equilibrium of animals, insects, and microorganisms in your garden so that parasites have no chance to multiply out of proportion. More than any green area, an herb garden is self-protective in that respect because of the conglomeration of so many intense aromas.

Finally, we wish you lots of fun and great success in planning, building, and starting your own herb garden!

Plants for the Herb Garden

Angelica	Angelica archangelica	Linden	Tilia platyphyllos
Balm	Melissa officinalis		Tilia cordata
Blackberry	Rubus fruticosus	Mallow	Malva sylvestris
		Marigold	Calendula officinalis
Caraway	Carum carvi	Melilot	Melilotus officinalis
Centaury	Centaurium erythraea	Mullein	Verbascum
Chamomile	Matricaria		densiflorum
	chamomilla		
	Chamomilla romana	Nettle, stinging	Urtica dioica
Chervil	Anthriscum		
	cerefolium	Onion	Allium cepa
Chive	Allium	Orange	Citrus aurantium
	schoenoprasum	Origanum	Origanum mayorana
Comfrey	Symphytum officinale		Origanum
Cone-flower	Echinacea		heracleoticum
	angustifolia		Origanum hirtum
	Echinacea purpurea		Origanum onites
	Echinacea pallida	Parsley	Petroselinum crispum
Dandelion	Taraxacum officinale	Plantain	Plantago lanceolata
Dill	Anethum graveolens	Peppermint	Mentha piperata
			Mentha aquatica
Elder	Sambucus niger	Pimpinella	Pimpinella saxifraga
			Pimpinella major
Fennel	Foeniculum vulgare		
Feverfew	Chrysanthemum	Raspberry	Rubus idaeus
	parthenium	Rose	Rosa
Flax	Linum usitatissimum	———, wild	Rosa canina
		Rosemary	Rosmarinus officinalis
Garlic	Allium sativum	Sage	Salvia officinalis
———, wild	Allium ursinum		Salvia montana
Geranium,		St. Johnswort	Hypericum
scented	Geranium odoratum		perforatum
Goldenrod	Solidago virgaurea	Strawberry, wild	Fragaria vesca
Hawthorn	Crataegus monogyna	Spearmint	Menta spicata
Hop	Humulus lupulus	Tarragon, French	Artemisia dracunculus
Horsetail	Equisetum arvense	Thyme	Thymus vulgaris
			Thymus zygis
Iris	Iris	Valerian	Valeriana officinalis
Juniper	Juniperus communis	Willow-herb	Epilobium
Lady's mantle	Alchemilla vulgaris		parviflorum
Laurelberry	Laurus nobilis	Yarrow	Achillea millefolium
Lavender	Lavandula		
	angustifolia		

BIBLIOGRAPHY

Airola, Paavo. *How to Get Well.* Phoenix: Health Plus, 1974.

Bollingen Foundation Inc., N.Y. *Paracelsus: Selected Writings.* Princeton, N.J.: Princeton University Press, 1973.

Bruker, M. O. *Krank durch Zucher* [Ill through sugar]. 7th ed. Bad Homburg: Schnitzer Verlag, 1978.

———. *Schicksal aus der Küche.* [Fate from the kitchen] *Zivilisationskrankheiten-Ursachen, Verhütung, Heilung* [Illnesses of civilization—their causes, prevention, and cure]. 7th ed. St. Georgen: Schnitzer Verlag, 1978.

Hochschild, Arlie, and Anne Machung. *The Second Shift: Inside the Two-Job Marriage.* New York: Viking, 1988.

Hoffmann, David. *The Herbal Handbook.* Rochester, Vt.: Healing Arts Press, 1988.

Peters, U. H., and K. Pollak. *Vom Kopfschmerz kann man sich befreien* [One can free oneself from headaches]. Munich: 1967.

Thie, John F. *Touch for Health.* Marina del Rey, Ca.; 1973.

Tompkins, P., and C. Bird. *The Secret Life of Plants.* New York: Harper & Row, 1984.

Treben, Maria. *Health from God's Pharmacy.* Steyr: Ennsthaler, 1980.

———. *Health from God's Garden.* Rochester, Vt.: Healing Arts Press, 1988.

Weiß, R. F. *Lehrbuch der Phytotherapie* [Textbook of phytotherapy]. Stuttgart: Hippokrates, 1985.

SUGGESTED READING

American Botanical Council. *HerbalGram*. Austin, Tx.

Becker, H., and H. Schmoll. *Mistel—Arzneipflanze, Brauchtum, Kunstmotiv im Jugendstil* [Mistletoe—medicinal plant, folklore, and art motif in Art Nouveau]. Stuttgart: Wissenschaftliche Verlagsgesellschaft, 1986.

Brucker, M. O. *Stuhlverstopfung heilbar—ohne Abführmittel* [Cure constipation without laxatives]. Lahnstein: Schnitzer Verlag, 1986.

Buchinger, Dr. O. *Heil-Fastenkur.* Hannover O. J.: Verlag H. Wilkens.

Bundesgesundheitsamt, Berlin. *Abwehr von Arzneimittelrisiken. Stufe II, Pyrrolizidinalkaloidhatige Humanarzneimittel* [Defense of risks caused by medications, Step II, Pyrrolizidine alkaloid–containing medications for human use]. Az. GV 7-7251-01-25365 Decree from 10.8.1988.

Chaitow, Leon, D. O., N. D. *Candida Albicans—Could Yeast Be Your Problem?* Rochester, Vt.: Healing Arts Press, 1987.

Christopher, John. *School of Natural Healing.* Provo, Ut.: Biworld, 1976.

Dawson, Adele G. *Herbs: Partners in Life.* Rochester, Vt.: Healing Arts Press, 1991.

de Bairacli Levy, Juliette. *The Illustrated Herbal Handbook.* London: Faber and Faber, 1982.

———. *Nature's Children* (out of print).

Deutsche Apotheker Zeitung, 132: 45, 5.11.1992 "Pharmazeutische Biologie, Pyrrolizidinalkaloidhaltige Arzneipflanzen" [Pharmaceutical biology of pyrrolizidine alkaloid–containing medications].

Diamond, Harvey, and Marilyn Diamond. *Fit for Life.* New York: Warner Books, 1987.

Elliott, Douglas B. *Roots: An Underground Botany and Forager's Guide.* Old Greenwich, Conn.: Chatman Press, 1976.

Foster, Steven. *Echinacea: Nature's Immune Enhancer.* Rochester, Vt.: Healing Arts Press, 1991.

———, and Yue Chongxi. *Herbal Emissaries: Bringing Chinese Herbs to the West.* Rochester, Vt.: Healing Arts Press, 1992.

Fulder, Steven. *The Book of Ginseng: Chinese Herbs for Immune Power.* Rochester, Vt.: Healing Arts Press, 1994.

Gladstar, Rosemary. *Herbal Healing for Women.* New York: Simon & Schuster, 1993.

Green, James. *The Male Herbal, Health Care for Men and Boys.* Freedom, Calif: Crossing Press, 1991.

Grieve, M. *A Modern Herbal.* Vol. I and II. New York: Dover Publications, 1971.

Griggs, Barbara. *Green Pharmacy: The History and Evolution of Western Herbal Medicine.* Rochester, Vt.: Healing Arts Press, 1991.

Hoffman, David. *An Elder's Herbal: Natural Techniques for Promoting Health and Vitality.* Rochester, Vt.: Healing Arts Press, 1991.

———. *The Holistic Herbal.* Findhorn, U.K.: Findhorn Press, 1988.

Holzner, Wolfgang. *Das kritische Heilpflanzen-Handbuch* [The critical herbal handbook]. Vienna: Orac, 1985

Hoppe, H. *Drogenkunde* [Textbook of dried herbs]. Vol. I and II, 8th ed. Berlin, New York: Walter de Gruyter, 1975.

Hutchens, Alma R. *Indian Herbology of North America.* London: The Garden City Press Limited, 1974.

Isaac, Otto. *Die Ringelblume* [The marigold]. Stuttgart: Wissenschaftliche Verlagsgesellschaft mbH, 1992.

Kaufmann, Klaus. *Silica: The Amazing Gel.* Burnaby, Canada: Alive Books, 1993.

Kloss, Jethro. *Back to Eden.* Loma Linda, Calif.: Back to Eden Books, 1982.

Künzle, Johann. *Das Grosse Kräuterheilbuch* [The great book of healing herbs]. Olten: Verlag Otto Walter AG, 1982.

Lützner, Helmut. *Wie neugeboren durch Fasten* [As new born through fasting]. Munich: Gräfe und Unzer, 1986.

———, and Helmut Million. *Richtig essen nach dem Fasten* [Eat right after a healing fast]. Munich: Gräfe und Unzer, 1992.

Mabey, Richard. *The New Age Herbalist.* New York: Collier Books/Macmillan, 1988.

Mills, Simon Y., M. A. *The Dictionary of Modern Herbalism.* Rochester, Vt.: Healing Arts Press, 1988.

Nissim, Rina. *Natural Healing in Gynecology.* New York: Pandora Press, 1986.

Pahlow, M. *Das große Buch der Heilpflanzen* [The great book of medicinal herbs]. Munich: Gräfe und Unzer, 1988.

Parvati, Jeannine. *Hygieia, A Woman's Herbal.* Monroe, Ut.: Freestone Press, 1978.

Petkov, V. D., and A. H. Mosharrof. "Effects of standardized ginseng extract on learning, memory and physical capabilities." *American Journal of Chinese Medicine* 15 (1987):19–29.

Revers, W. J., et al. "Psychological effects of a geriatric preparation in the aged." *Zeitschrift für präklinische und klinische Geriatrie* 6 (1976):418–430.

Riggs, Maribeth. *Natural Child Care.* New York: Crown, 1988.

Rose, Jeanne. *Herbs and Things.* New York: Grosset and Dunlap, 1969.

Schilcher, H. "Pflanzliche Diuretika" [Phyto-diuretics]. *Zeitschrift für Phyto-therapie,* No. 5, Stuttgart, 1987.

Schneider, H.-J. "Therapie und Metaphylaxe der Urolithiasis mit Phyto-pharmaka, *Zeitschrift für Phytotherapie,* No. 5, Stuttgart, 1987.

Schultes, Richard Evans, and Albert Hofmann. *Plants of the Gods: Their Sacred, Healing, and Hallucinogenic Powers.* Rochester, Vt.: Healing Arts Press, 1992.

Simonton, O. Carl, S. Matthews-Simonton, and J. Creighton. *Getting Well Again.* New York: Bantam, 1978.

Stammel, H. J. *Die Apotheke Manitous* [Manitou's apothecary]. Reinbeck: Wunderlich, 1986.

Storl, Wolf-Dieter. *Der Garten als Mikrokosmos.* Freiburg im Breisgau: Hermann Bauer Verlag KG, 1882.

Tesch, P. A., et al. "The effect of ginseng, vitamins and minerals on the physical work capacity in middle-aged men." *Läkartidningen* 84 (1987):4326–4328.

Theiss, P., and B. Theiss. *Neue Lebenskraft durch Heilkräuter* [New life energy through medicinal herbs]. Homburg-Saar: Self-publication, 1981.

Tierra, Lesley. *The Herbs of Life.* Freedom, Ca.: Crossing Press, 1992.

Tierra, Michael. *The Way of Herbs.* New York: Simon & Schuster, 1990.

Trowbridge, John Parks, M.D., and Morton Walker, D.P.M. *The Yeast Syndrome.* New York: Bantam Books, 1986.

Tyler, Varro E., Ph.D. *The New Honest Herbal.* Philadelphia: George F. Stickley Company, 1987.

Weed, Susun. *The Wise Woman Herbal for the Childbearing Years.* Woodstock, N.Y.: Ash Tree Publishing, 1986.

———. *Wise Woman Herbal for the Menopausal Years.* Woodstock, N.Y.: Ash Tree Publishing, 1992.

Wichtl, M. *Teedrogen, Ein Handbuch für die Praxis auf wissenschaftlicher Grundlage* [A handbook for practice on a scientific basis], 2nd ed. Stuttgart: Wissenschlaftliche Verlagsgesellschaft, 1989.

Zuin, M., et al. "Effects of a preparation containing a standardized ginseng extract combined with trace elements and multivitamins against hepa-totoxin-induced chronic liver disease in the elderly." *Journal of International Medical Research* 15 (1987):276–281.

HERBAL SUPPLIERS

Your local health food store or herbal supply should carry most of the items mentioned in this book. You might also want to refer to the following list of wholesale suppliers.

UNITED STATES

NatureWorks
5341 Derry Ave.
Agoura Hills, CA
91301

(NatureWorks wholesales most of the supplies and herbs mentioned in this book).

Merz Apothecary
4716 N. Lincoln Ave.
Chicago, IL 60625

(This company can fulfill retail mail orders for most of the supplies and herbs mentioned in this book).

Aphrodesia Products, Inc.
62 Kent St.
Brooklyn, NY 11201

Frontier Co-op Herbs
Box 299
Norway, IA 52318

Star and Crescent Herbs
8551 Thys Ct., Suite C
Sacramento, CA 95828

Taylor's Herb Gardens
1535 Lone Oak Rd.
Vista, CA 92084

Turtle Island Herbs
Salina Star Route
Boulder, CO 80302

Yerba Prima
P.O. Box 2569
Oakland, CA 94614

CANADA

Purity Life Health Products
100 Elgin St. South
Acton, Ontario
Canada L7J 2W1

Flora Distributors
7400 Fraser Park Drive
Burnaby, B.C.
Canada V5J 5B0

AUSTRALIA

International Health
    Promotions
7/39 Herbert St.
St. Leonards
New South Wales 2065
Australia

NEW ZEALAND

Wagner Pro Biotics Ltd.
112 Gill St.
P.O. Box 4142
New Plymouth
New Zealand

SWEDEN

Sol Tryck
Rörbergvägen
81800 Valbo
Sweden

MALAYSIA

Nature's Herbs SDN. BHD.
No. 40 1st Floor, Jalan SS 2/66
47300 Petaling Jaya
Selangor D.E.
West Malaysia

NIGERIA

Starling Nigeria Ltd.
17, Alhaji Tokan St.
Surulere, Lagos
Nigeria

USEFUL ADDRESSES

American Botanical Council
P.O. Box 201660
Austin, TX 78720

American Herbal Products
Association (AHPA)
P.O. Box 2410
Austin, TX 78768

Herb Research Foundation
1007 Pearl St., Suite 200
Boulder, CO 80302
(Tel: 303-449-2265)

PLANT INDEX

Listed in this section of the index are the forty major herbs discussed in the book. All other herbs are listed in the second section of the index. Page numbers in *bold italic* type refer to principal references and/or photographs of plants.

❧ BOTANICAL NAMES ❧

INDEX